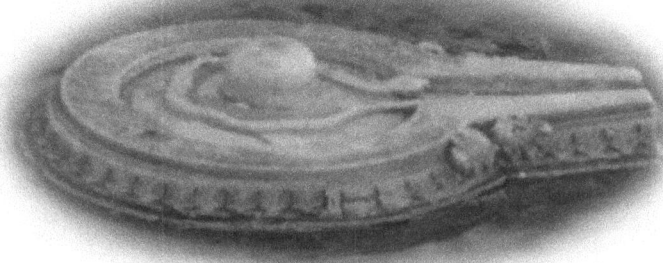

IYAM YONIH SAMĀKHYĀTĀ
SARVATANTRESHU SARVADĀ /
CATURDASHAYUTAM BHADRE TITHĪSHĀNTA
SAMANVITAM // 9

इयं योनिः समाख्याता सर्वतन्त्रेषु सर्वदा ।
चतुर्दशयुतं भद्रे तिथीशान्तसमन्वितम् ॥ ९ ॥

"This *yoni* is filled with the 'shining forth' of the four illustrious
elements in balance with the expansive world."

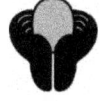

The Mystical Shiva Linga
Lingam (*masculine*)
Yoni (*feminine*)
Serpent (*evolution*)

T he ancient *Shiva Linga* Icon shown in the Frontispiece, along with the sacred writings called the *Vedas*, are the principal and nearly the only artifacts left behind by the ancient Aryans who invaded the Indus Valley several millennia before the Christian era. There is no doubt that both the Icon and the *Vedas* contain a powerful secret related to creation and personal powers. Yet the secret has remained largely hidden over the millennia following the Aryans.

The *Sanskrit* verse shown on the Frontispiece is from a recently uncovered and translated text that describes the *yoni* (symbolized in the Icon) as the source of a creative power. The full text describes how the three elements of the Icon can be found within you and used to create new worlds. The power of the *yoni* is also described as the mythical elixir called *soma*, the central theme of the *Vedas*.

The Triune of the three elements of the Icon and in the newly translated text suggested the title for this book, The Golden Triangle.

The Golden Triangle

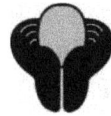

ROBERT LESTER PECK

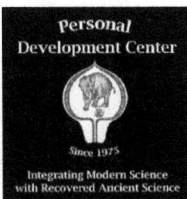

Personal
Development Center

Since 1975

Integrating Modern Science
with Recovered Ancient Science

PERSONAL
DEVELOPMENT CENTER LLC
Lebanon, Connecticut U.S.A. 1998

www.personaldevcenter.com

3 4 5 6 7 8 9 10

Publisher's Note

This third printing, November 2025, of the original 1998 publication of *The Golden Triangle* contains format changes. The margins and font sizes of the text were reduced, and the font of *The Emerald Tablet* was changed. All previous changes made in the second September 2022 printing remain the same. (i.e. minor editorial corrections throughout the text, format improvements, an added index, a correction of the title *The Emerald Table* to *The Emerald Tablet*, and the Frontispiece adjustment to include the author's translation of the *Sanskrit* verse.)

Translations of Greek terms and *Sanskrit* terms of the *Parātriṃshikā* (Thirty Verses), The Sermon on the Mount, and the *Sanskrit Tantrik* dictionary are by Robert Lester Peck (a.k.a. Robert L. Peck) unless otherwise noted. In addition, the data compiled in the Figures and/or Tables in *The Greatest Medical Myth* section of the book were compiled for this publication by Robert L. Peck.

Cover design by Lois Rivard.

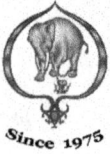

Personal Development Center
P.O. Box 93
South Windham, Connecticut 06266-0093

Since 1975   ©1998 Robert L. Peck

ISBN 13: 978-0917828-06-5 (Paperback)
ISBN 10: 0-917828-06-2 (Paperback)

ISBN 13: 978-0917828-20-1 (eBook)
ISBN 10: 0-917828-20-8 (eBook)

Printed in the United States of America

TABLE OF CONTENTS

PREFACE

The writing of this book is supported by the discovery and translation of an ancient *Sanskrit* document called the *Parātrimshikā*. The author found the *Parātrimshikā* in an eleventh century Indian document called the *Parātrīsikā Vivaraṇa* (Note spelling difference of the middle syllables of "*trim*" vs "*tris*") written by the Indian sage and mystic, Abhinavagupta. The *Parātrīsikā Vivaraṇa* was an extension and commentary on the much older *Parātrimshikā* which probably was based on oral traditions going back to or preceding the Indian *Vedas*, *Āgamas* and *Tantras*, the world's oldest religious writings.

The formidable *Parātrīsikā Vivaraṇa* was written to expound upon the *Parātrimshikā* that is contained within it. However, as you read the *Parātrīsikā Vivaraṇa* more closely, you discover that it is really a tutorial upon the concepts required to understand the inner text. Over twenty percent of this interesting mystical book is spent in telling the reader how to dissect and manipulate the *Sanskrit* terms to properly translate the much older inner document. The genius of Abhinavagupta can be understood as he uses a surface translation of the *Parātrimshikā* to explain the complex system of the *Tantrik* model of the mystical body and mind.

The meaning of the inner document is still hidden, however, even with the assistance from Abhinavagupta. This is because the inner document speaks of processes that will be interpreted wrongly if they have not been experienced. Without that experience, you can only rely upon the commentary, which is very complex and difficult to follow with a science foreign to the modern world. Modern references to this writing claim it to be one of India's most challenging books to read. The *Parātrimshikā* can best be described as a very scientific or technical writing, and like any other technical writing it is meaningful only to those who have been initiated into the specialized nomenclature and teachings.

The *Parātrimshikā*, in summary, was written for that one person in a thousand spoken of as one of the "select" in religious writings. If the reader has not experienced the higher realms or sensations that were written about, the document becomes a meaningless and obtuse manuscript. However, if you are curious, open and willing to explore, then you will be fascinated with this strange document and feel that something great is contained within it. The obscurity of the writing can also be explained in that it was written for the *Kaliyuga* or the "Age of Darkness" to preserve the ancient wisdom for the dawning of a better time.

This book is intended to be primarily a modern extension of the contents of the *Parātrīśikā Vivaraṇa*, with support from other ancient writings, as well as a source of modern scientific wisdom. *The Golden Triangle* reveals much of the philosophy and practices as well as other material assumed to have been taught by the ancient sages. *The Golden Triangle* is written in the same technical style as the earlier writings, and hence is not academic with each statement limited or supported by the normal outside authoritative references. Rather, it is written to be self-supportive in that the preceding statements as well as personal experiential verification supports each new statement. If this is not found to be true, then this book may not be for you or you need to restudy the prior discussions. Statements cannot be taken out of context nor read out of order. Further, the reading of the whole document is necessary for understanding, since all of the statements are interconnected. References to authoritative books are given in the Appendix if you care to investigate further.

The *Parātrimshikā* discusses a super power that resides within the *hridaya*, "heart" or "center-of-self" located between the thighs. This power is associated with strong feminine and androgynous characteristics that are maintained by the generation and flow of an inner creative fluid called *soma* (the mystical elixir of the *Vedas*). Because it is the source of powers, knowledge, and ecstasy of living, this center provides a connection directly to Heaven. The opening of this heart is reached through what is called *mātrena* or the union of the "Sun" and "Moon." Upon opening the heart, one finds the mystical gifts and powers described by the world's major religions as well the very physical forces utilized by the original martial arts. The Sun, Moon and created Heaven which constitute the basis of *The Golden Triangle* are found to have been at one time universal and expressed in many ways throughout the world.

The Golden Triangle was written for you if you are an active, creative person who has experienced inexplicable changes in your mind and body that include six or more of the following:

    a.   Inexplicable pleasurable sexual-like or upward rushes of feelings.

b. Sensations of an increased opening or sensitivity of the perineum.

c. Feelings of being androgynous or having opposite sex characteristics.

d. Perceiving the nature of the world as different from what you were taught.

e. Increased faith in your own goals in life or a sense that your dedications are coming to fruition.

f. Pressures in the head and chest initiated with slight or subtle emotions.

g. Strengthened drive to understand the self and life.

h. Increased awareness of inner ringing of the ear (tinnitus) or in the head.

i. Some ability to intentionally change your world and how you feel.

j. Moments of transcendence in levels of awareness or consciousness.

k. Increased sense of softness, tenderness toward others or more people.

l. Increased desire to have more intimacy (non-sexual) with others.

m. Feelings of not belonging and being separated from others.

The contents of this book are also the result of an extensive verification of the esoteric models and practices by several large groups of volunteer middle-class Americans (without any exchange of money). These people were willing to attempt to undergo and evaluate each exercise or practice to determine its fitness and value in today's world. After twenty years of research and practices, it was concluded that participants would find changes in the physiology of the body and increases in mental capabilities that agree in general with those mentioned in ancient writings. It also became evident that another mode of presentation of these practices was required for the modern age and that the participants' efforts also helped to produce those modes of presentation.

The author wishes to honor the traditions of India that maintained, preserved and revered the ancient documents without burning, destroying, or excessively modifying them as was commonly done in Western history.

The author also pays homage to the early sages and teachers who wrote in such a remarkable manner that their Truths could be discerned in the modern world. Also, this book could not have materialized without the continual dedication of those supportive people seeking to explore the relevancy of the ancient writings to today's world. The author also honors the couples who meticulously worked and experimented with the *yoni* couplings of *maithuna* and reported their findings. The author offers his thanks to these generous people and to their faith that the ancient truths could be enlivened in the midst of the marketplace of our materialistic society.

There were also some highly dedicated people who sacrificed much in supporting the finalizing of this book and its preparation for publishing. These people chose to remain anonymous even though this book could not have materialized without their efforts.

The teachings of this book evidence the true source.

Note: This book will italicize the *Sanskrit* (*Sáṃskṛita*) terms and list their meaning in the *Sanskrit*-to-English Dictionary in the Appendix. For those with some knowledge of *Sanskrit*, the original *Parātriṃshikā* in *Sanskrit* (English transliteration) is printed in Chapter Fifteen.

WARNING

The disciplines in this book work with the interaction of the body and mind. The body can be stimulated, for instance, to increase sensory perception, strength, sensitivity, and the power to give reality to the constructs of the mind. If the body is stimulated without the necessary mental controls, the mind can become deeply depressed, fearful, or aggressive. Similarly, if the mind is developed without the necessary physical development, the body can become more stimulated than it can withstand, resulting in severe damage and possible death. As an example, imagine placing your present mind in the body of a child, or the mind of a child within your body.

You should be careful in seeking personal assistance. Masters of the spiritual path do not profit from their services, and the reader should avoid seeking assistance from anyone who requires a fee or donation for guidance. Since the results of the included practices are systemic, any Master should be able to explain all of your symptoms or problems based only on a few interrogative questions or observations. No Master needs to revert to any further analysis. Do not entrust yourself to the guidance of anyone who has not directly experienced your level of development as well as the higher levels.

THE ANCIENT MYSTICAL TEXTS

1

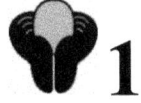

AN INTRODUCTION

T he *Golden Triangle* recovers some of the keys to the powers described in the ancient writings by the discovery and translation of a very ancient *Sanskrit* document called the *Parātriṃshikā* or the *Thirty Transcending Statements*. These thirty concise maxims, which date back long before the Christian era, do in fact open unknown doors that can lead you into the ecstasy and powers of life promised by so many of the world's mystical and religious writings.

The first invaluable contribution of the *Parātriṃshikā* is the presentation of some basic and very surprising definitions of terms used in many of the old writings. Without these proper definitions, it is easy to see how so much confusion about and misuse of the old religious and philosophical writings and teachings prevail today. For instance, consider your present definitions and feelings about the basic religious words: "heaven," "heart" and "spirit." You no doubt find these terms vague and abstract with little relationship to your daily life. As will be shortly demonstrated, the *Parātriṃshikā* defines these terms as relating to definite places and forces that exist within or emanate out of the lower abdominal region of your body, controlled by an almost unknown yet physically manifest organ which requires specific exercises for its full development.

As a brief introduction, "Heaven" as used in the old texts is not a place of your afterlife. Your "heart" is in fact the center of your existence, but is not in the head or chest. "Spirit" refers to an indwelling and controllable power that lies behind the supernormal and largely unexplained feats accomplished by individuals. The amazing *Parātriṃshikā* provides the long-lost definitions of many of these mystical terms used around the world and provides the clues for finding a deeper understanding of many of the early writings and claims of Alchemy, the martial arts, *Yoga*, the *Tao*, Christianity as well as other mystical writings. With accurate definitions, the difference between the religious, mystical, and scientific fields also diminishes. It will also be shown that science is really built upon the ancient mystical four elements with a viewpoint of energy that is compatible with the forefront of modern physics today. Modern physiology and psychology have "thrown the baby out with the bath water" in by-

1

passing subjective feelings. Instead of finding feelings subjective, the ancient Masters found many of them to be definitely objective physiological changes as will be discussed.

Another contribution of the *Parātriṃshikā* to the modern age is to point to the universality of the ancient writings. As an example, the meaning of the "One becoming Two" (a Creator starting with the creation of two items) is found in nearly the same wording in the *Parātriṃshikā* of Northern India, the *Tao Te Ching* of China, and *The Emerald Tablet* of ancient Egypt. The "Two" is also generally described as the "Sun and Moon" or as an equivalent the "Masculine and Feminine." The "Two" also has two locations, either in the Heavens above or within you. It is the indwelling "Sun and Moon" that provide the powers to transform your world.

Another important teaching to be gained from the *Parātriṃshikā* is that many of the important ancient mystical documents were written as technical discourses that intended to elucidate important concepts rather than to simply inspire or preach. As technical writings, they can be compared to modern papers written on physics, psychology, chemistry, or other technical subjects that require a prior knowledge of the technical terms and their usage. Another important requirement of technical papers is that there must be a step-by-step reading of the text. You cannot take isolated statements out of text or attempt to randomly read the text out of order by skipping unintelligible paragraphs.

Perhaps the most startling aspects of the *Parātriṃshikā* are its references to androgyny as a necessity for evolution or transcendence. The *Parātriṃshikā* describes the center of androgyny as being within the *yoni*. This connection clarifies the classical writings of *Yoga* which describe the location and activity of a *yoni* although generally misunderstood as being the female pudenda. It is also apparent upon reflection that androgyny appears in many of the world's early religious writings. For instance, many writings speak of sexual changes before ascending to higher realms. The union with the Divine is often described as entering into a sexual tryst with the Divine with a sexual role reversal. Another interesting point is that the traditional Priests from many religions can be identified because of the feminine nature of their garb. The source of this custom is no doubt long forgotten.

The *Parātriṃshikā* identifies the source of androgyny as resulting from the union of your inner Sun and Moon. This Sun and Moon in their union create your personal Heaven or perfected world. The inner Sun, Moon, and inner Heaven constitute a Trinity that corresponds to another external Trinity of Sun, Moon, and Earth. The ancient esoteric or secret powers lay in the control of the inner Sun and Moon and this was done in part by stimulating their dwelling place in the *yoni*.

The thirty statements of the *Parātriṃshikā* when combined with the extant mystical teachings, modern science, and experimental verifications form the basis of *The Golden Triangle*. The original philosophies taught that there is an underlying spiritual formation that precedes the physical manifestation of everything that you experience. This means that there is a real aspect of *entelechy* or directed and defined will power that must be addressed if you truly desire to find change or evolution in your daily life. However, to change your world and Self, there likewise must be a change within the physical body and its chemistry in order to connect the physical with the subtle or spiritual realms. This change corresponds to the rapid changes taking place in prepubescent children that, as will be discussed, are associated with intense lower abdominal activity. Although this activity is suppressed by our society as children mature, some adults can remember the strong sexual-like feelings associated with this state of the body and the associated zest, fervor, and passion for life. Many of the monastic-type practices used around the world loosen the abdominal tensions and mental controls gained in growing to adulthood such that the creative energy of childhood can be reclaimed.

The Emerald Tablet

It is true,
that as it is above, so it is below.
All things are from the One,
by the One becoming Two.

The Sun is the Father, the Mother is the Moon.
The breath has carried it to the belly
and the body nurtures.

The gateway to perfection is now opened
through this potential
lying in the depths of the physical.
Only with the greatest care,
is the physical separated from the subtle
or the subtle from the physical.

It rises from the depths to the heights;
descends, while the higher and lower
magnify the power.

The promise is as follows:
The world in all its glory
is seen with clarity and wisdom.
More powerful than strength and force,
solid and subtle are conquered,
and thus all is created, that which is,
and the perfection of tomorrow.

From Hermes Trismegistus, 1st Century

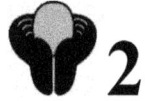

TWO ANCIENT DOCUMENTS
The Emerald Tablet ~ The Parātriṃshikā

One of the oldest (first Century AD) and most revered writings on the arcane science of Alchemy is *The Emerald Tablet*[1] written by the legendary father of Alchemy, Hermes Trismegistus (Messenger of the Three Powers). *The Emerald Tablet* survived through the ages because as brief as it is, it has a strong impact on most readers as somehow touching upon some very important truth. For the majority of people, Alchemy has been perceived as a route to fabulous material wealth through the conversion of lead to gold and this no doubt kept the writings from being burned. A much smaller number of people, however, perceive it as a possible guide to the perfection of the Self and it is for these few people that many of the ancient documents and this book were written.

Several beginning exemplary comparisons can be made between the "conversion" processes spoken of by the Alchemists and by the early Christians (not related to today's usage of the word "conversion"). The Alchemists described their reaction vessel in which the conversion took place as the "athanor" similar in shape and size to the human body. The athanor can also be compared with the water vessels of similar size described in the Wedding at Cana in the Bible. Alchemy used the infusion of "immortal fire" or *ignis innaturalis* into the athanor, while Christianity describes the conversion process by the infusion of "Spirit" into the water vessels for the conversion of water into wine. (Indian models used a similar model with *soma* as will be discussed later.) The Alchemists describe the end result of the conversion process as pure refined gold, whereas the Christians describe it as vintage wine. The use of wine (or leavened bread) was an allegorical term characteristic of the early Western philosophers. This usage was based upon their belief that the conversion of grapes (or flour) into a higher form could be compared to the change in individuals as they opened to a Divine Spirit.

---

[1] See page 5.

One characteristic of early religious writings is that they contain two or more levels of understanding. The upper level or most widely understood level was generally politically correct for its time or was acceptable to the majority of people. The lower or hidden levels were only understood by a small percentage of readers who would be those few who had "ears to hear" as described by Jesus. If you have the "ears to hear" you can perceive the two levels of writing in the story of the Wedding at Cana. The average person desires magical powers and only reads the story as depicting super powers that would impress their friends. If, however, the readers are seeking union with a higher power or the joy of life, then they see the transformation of water in the water vessels as an allegory for the infusion of some transformational "Spirit" within their own bodies or the injection of a higher state of consciousness into themselves. This hidden level of teaching refers to the greatest of miracles which far exceeds the magic of making wine.

In unraveling the "secrets" of the ancient writings, it must be under-stood that these were not secrets but rather "truths" to those individuals who had already mastered their social world and had some experiences with their inner vital forces and processes. These ancient writings were, however, veiled and misdirecting to those who were seeking power, gold, wine and sex. To those individuals, the writings became sacred and were worshiped as a potential source for satisfying their lusts. If this element had not been written into the documents they might not have survived, particularly if they were to be preserved by greedy or power-hungry institutional leaders.

Before proceeding on, it is helpful to also mention again that many of the original mystical writings were very technical in nature. This means that the ancients were careful to define their terms that were inserted into the text. You cannot take a line or verse out of context in these writings since all of the thoughts must build upon and be consistent with the others. (All of the points being raised will be discussed in detail later, but it would be timely for the reader who likes to jump about in a book to be patient and recognize the importance of the "step-by-step" or *krama* process described by the early writers. This will become evident with later detailed discussions of some of the writings.)

The Emerald Tablet will be used as a general outline for the beginning of this book since it is compatible with the Western mind and models. *Part A* of this book will therefore set the stage for the understanding of what is meant by the separation of the subtle from the physical or the Sun from the Moon. *Part B* is based upon the author's translation of a hidden Indian document called the *Parātriṃshikā* which is probably as old as the *Vedas* or created before 500 BC. This document is very similar to *The Emerald Tablet* in pointing toward an inner power, yet it goes beyond the Alchemical document by discussing how the Sun and Moon once separated can be reunited to create Heavens. This compares to the second half of the Alchemical reaction (not described in *The Emerald Tablet*) which involves recombining the separated elements to create "gold."

In India a few discourses have been written about the *Parātriṃshikā* including two by Abhinavagupta, an eleventh century writer who is often quoted by those exploring *Tantra*. It is interesting that Abhinavagupta did not offer a direct translation of the *Parātriṃshikā* but did write about how it could be done, which made the translation possible for the author of this book. His commentaries are similar to those on Alchemy in that they do not directly address the esoteric teachings, but do offer insights and guideposts for those who are seeking and are ready for them.

In order to prepare you for the *Parātriṃshikā* and how it can be used to unravel the hidden teachings, a brief comparison between it and *The Emerald Tablet* will be given. Each verse of *The Emerald Tablet* is given with a corresponding selected verse from the *Parātriṃshikā*. The complete *Parātriṃshikā* is given in Chapter Fifteen with the literal translation as well as summary comments. The transliterated *Sanskrit* is included as well for the serious *Sanskrit* student to follow.

The terms and their meanings, which are obtained by the careful step-by-step analysis of the documents, will be described in detail in later chapters, but to simplify the initial reading, a few of the resulting critical definitions are listed below.[2]

Sun and **Moon**: The universal symbols for the Masculine and Feminine such as the *Yang* and *Yin* of the Chinese or the unmanifest and manifest natures or forces. Personified in many religions as an indwelling God and Goddess (in the Heaven described below).

---

[2] A more complete *Sanskrit* Dictionary is given in the Appendix.

Hridayam: as the center of action or of life and not the beating heart in
    Hridaya: Heart the chest. The *hridaya* is located within
    the sexual region or in the lower belly of the body.

Mantra: The intentional mental creation or conative process.

Mudrā: The manifesting of that mental creation or *mantra*.

Tantra: The advanced *Yoga* system dealing with the inner energies of
    the body.

Shiva: An indwelling God and the source of the masculine powers.

Heaven: The highest state of existence of *anuttara*. It is the
    same as the Bible's term of the kingdom of Heaven "within"
    you and is not a future place after death.

As a starting comparison of *The Emerald Tablet* and the *Parātriṃshikā*, each statement of *The Emerald Tablet* is listed below with selected verses from the *Parātriṃshikā*. The first statement of each paragraph is from *The Emerald Tablet* in normal bold print, while the immediately following verse(s) in italics are from the *Parātriṃshikā* with the number of the verse included. Because of the intercomparison, the verses of the *Parātriṃshikā* are not given in order.

Of this it is certain,
that as it is above, so it is below.
All things are from the One,
by the One becoming Two.
The Sun is the Father, the Mother is the Moon.

All of the reality of Heaven can be found to be built on; and becomes manifest with the subtle union of the Moon and Sun. //5

**The breath has carried it to the belly
and the body nurtures.**

*This hridayam in the belly is the dwelling place of the God of gods
and is the source of union with liberation at the same time. //11*

*The illustrious feminine power is the source of the great Divine
gifts in the kingdom of Heaven. //3*

**The gateway to perfection is now opened through this
potential lying in the depths of the physical.**

*By maintaining Tantrik practices, the desired world is made real,
thrust forth from the Heaven within your heart (hridaya). //4*

*The third sexual nature or the heart between the thighs unites the
Soul with the Divine. Those who do not have the state of androgyny
cannot break forth. //10*

**Only with the greatest care,
is the physical separated from the subtle or
the subtle from the physical.**

*The physical or manifest is in union with the Creative in the
developing world. Evolution proceeds step-by-step from one realm to
another. //6*

*At that time, one attains the empirical form of the mantra-mudrā,
that was created in the future and became manifest in the present. //13*

**It rises from the depths to the heights; descends, while the
higher and lower magnify the power.**

*The junction of the two brings forth all of the powers in the form of
a flowing unseen creative fluid. //18*

At the moment of opening, the body moves expressing the union with a continuing expression and enjoyment of sensual and ecstatic up-flowing feelings associated with a mudrā. //12

**The world in all its glory
is seen with clarity and wisdom.**

Because of the radiant fluid one is a great Soul, knowing the masculine powers of Shiva and all things, one is without sin, one's Will and exertions become pure and shining. //24

More powerful than strength and force, solid and subtle are conquered, and thus all is created.

As the great banyan tree is contained within the energy of its seed, so also is the evolutionary upper kingdom of Heaven contained as a seed in the hridaya. //25

This created power bursts forth from the combined masculine and feminine powers to attain all knowledge and powers. //30

The remaining chapters in this book will elaborate on these mystical documents by adding the ancient insights as to what constitutes life and the physical world, as well as describing the process for finding the kingdom of Heaven or perfection.

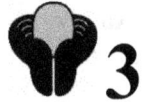

THE *ONE*, THE *TWO*, AND *TRINITY*

"All things are from the One, by the One becoming Two.
The Sun is the Father, the Mother is the Moon."
"As above, so below."

The Emerald Tablet

"and God divided the light from the darkness"

The Bible

T he ancient sages looked to the sky for their explanations or models of the creation and maintenance of the earth and its dwellers. As the sages formulated models of how the earth was created by the Heavens above, they found that these same models could also be allegories for what happened within their own personal manifest world. Many sages, as their experience and wisdom increased, discovered that the powers ascribed to the celestial objects were found to be powers within their own minds and bodies as will be presented in this and following chapters.

The statement from *The Emerald Tablet* about the "One" is an excellent starting point for the discussion of the early philosophies. The "One" according to *The Emerald Tablet* is the source or creator of the Sun and Moon that consequently became the creators of the earth. This concept of creation is almost universal in the major religions with the Sun and Moon being generally described as Masculine (Father) and Feminine (Mother) forces. Many of the ancient paintings depicting masculine gods or divine beings, portrayed their divinity with the disk or halo of the sun behind their heads while some of the feminine deities had a disk similar to the moon similarly placed behind their heads.

To approach the physical models used in the ancient writings, it is necessary to set aside much of modern wisdom and to see and feel the world with the senses. With this approach, it is obvious that the sun and moon rule the sky, but what the modern person forgets is that the sun and moon are both the exact same size (to the eyes). The size and nature of the sun and moon was determined during the solar eclipse when the moon exactly covered the face or surface of the sun and showed the outer ring of fire around the solar disk. The moon could be perceived as a solid disk (or possibly a ball) capable of hiding or covering the sun, while the sun appeared as a luminous disk of fire the same size as the moon. Since the two appeared the same size occupying the same sky, it was easy for the ancients to assume therefore, that originally the two were one, with the fire of the sun attached to and covering the moon. The fire may then be assumed to have dropped away earlier from the moon much as a ball of hot pitch will drop away from a burning stick and burst into flame as it falls. The sun and moon, therefore, can be considered to have come from the "One" and are two separate manifestations of the "One."

To the ancients the characteristics of the sun were quite obvious. The sun was vaporous without solidity, radiating heat and light similar to a flame. The sun controlled the seasons as well as the day and night. The sun was known to increase the creative power of the mind and increase awareness of the world and appeared to be the power source for life as well as for consciousness. Under the full power of the sun, the activity of life increased.

Unlike the ancients, the modern philosophers largely ignore the characteristics of the moon as well as its cyclical phases. Even the effect of the lunar month upon the menstrual cycle is forgotten and is minimized as the inner electrical lights at night in modern homes counter the varying intensity of the lunar light. The passive nurturing nature of the moon is also lost in the lights of the cities and homes. Many of the medical people report the strange effects of the full moon on the body and mind that were accepted as real to the ancients living under the moon. Whereas the sun appeared to control the cycles of nature, the moon was assumed to control the personal lives of humans and became the time clock for religious observations and special social events. Related to the social and personal timing was the height of the seas or the tides that resulted also from some hidden powers of the moon. Because of its passive, hidden yet personal powers, the moon was related to the universal feminine force while the dominating, driving, heating, creative powers of the sun were equated to the masculine nature.

In addition to perceiving the sun and moon as celestial powers, the ancients also observed five very strange and unique "stars" that wandered around the night sky seemingly independent of the rest of the stars marching in step across the night sky. These five "stars" we now know to be planets and in fact do appear to wander randomly through the sky each with its own unique path, brightness, or color. This uniqueness suggests individuality and freedom from the rigid disciplined motion of the multitude of stars. It would be natural for the ancients to contrive stories of these aberrant sources of light suggestive or symbolic of forces controlling those people below who did not march in unison with the majority of people through life.

Without elaborating on the powers associated with these wandering planets, it is important to mention that the forces or natures symbolized by them became fairly universal. It follows that the sun and the moon plus the five wanderers became the symbolic basis for seven unseen, unpredictable, and powerful forces affecting life. These forces or celestial objects were also symbolized by unpredictable anthropomorphic figures or gods who were easy to visualize. These seven forces, celestial bodies, or gods became the basis for the seven stages of individual attainment or evolution. As they were worshiped or appeased, they became associated with the seven days of the week. As an example, Sunday, or the day of the Sun became the day of worship of the creative source in many cultures. It was because of these seven celestial objects that the number seven took on mystical significance implying the full powers of the Celestial Heaven such as were used in many of the various apocalyptic or expositional religious writings.

The response of the people to this concept of the Celestial Powers took two routes. The first route led to the worship of these Powers in order to modify or change their life here below. This route led to the development of churches, temples, and priesthoods as intermediaries between the populace and the Celestial Heavenly Powers. The second route started with the recognition that some individuals appeared to have powers akin to those associated with the Celestial Heavenly Powers and were quite superior to others. In studying these accomplished individuals, it became clear that there were certain things or practices that these evolved people did which could be equated to the development of specific powers. These "things" were found to be universal and became the practices or *sādhanās* of *Tantra*.

This study therefore resulted in the acquiring of the wisdom about the forces and powers within the Self as well as the practices that enhanced or controlled them. This effort resulted in the development of the *Tantrik* systems as well as the later Alchemical, mystical and esoteric schools and

15

the following scientific disciplines such as Chemistry, Physics, Biology, etc. At the same time, there appeared another model of creation and control which centered itself within the individual rather than within the Celestial Heaven above. As will be discussed, as the Celestial Heaven above could create the physical world, so too could an inner Heaven within you create an outer experiential world that could also become a Heaven. The inner Heaven contained the equivalents of the celestial Sun and Moon.

One important philosophical point presented in the above model of the sun and moon is the creation of a dyad (two elements with opposite characteristics) from nothing or the "One." This creation of dyads can be used to explain the nature of bringing forth your own creations from nothing. It can be assumed that if the elements of a dyad are in fact true opposites, then when they are combined, they will equally interact together and annihilate each other leaving nothing. This resulting nothingness should therefore contain the combined two elements and hence, they should be able to be pulled forth later as two separate elements. As an example of this thinking, many theoretical physicists accept the concept of the existence of matter and anti-matter, which when brought together results in the annihilation of both. Another example is given with the Black Holes in space into which matter disappears.

The creation of the universe out of nothing by creating the matter/anti-matter dyad seems somewhat logical to explain where things came from. Heat pumps are another example. If heat is removed from a container of water at room temperature and put into another container of water also at room temperature, the first container of water becomes cold while the other becomes hot. If the two containers are then mixed together, the resultant temperature is the starting temperature of the first container. In this case, you may argue that you are creating heat and cold from something akin to the nothing. You might imagine a large tank of black paint that contains, of course, all colors that make it black. It is possible that you could remove the various colors with some filter or process which would give you many different colored paints which when remixed together later would result with the original black paint.

The Western world uses a dyad model similar to that of the sun and moon to explain your creation or existence. The Bible states that you are formed of two opposites: the spirit (Sun) that comes from God and dust (Moon) that comes from the earth. When you die, these elements return to their source as stated in the burial ceremonies of the West. It should be noted that it takes energy of the right type in all of the above examples to bring forth opposites from nothing, as will be explained later in regards to creating your own realities.

Creation can therefore proceed from nothing by the creation of opposites that would return to nothing or neutrality if brought together. This idea was expanded to include such dyads as: manifest and spiritual, life and death, hot and cold, light and dark, expansion and contraction, good and evil, positive and negative, etc. This expanded system of duality was named the "Two Truths" in early Egypt and served as the basis for many of the dualistic (*dvaita*) philosophical and religious developments.

Monism (*advaita*) or "Oneness" was based upon the primary consideration of the Nothingness from which the Dyads appeared. The Nothingness that can divide into opposing elements to create reality must originally have had the characteristics of the elements of the Dyads and hence cannot be truly nothing. Similarly, each element of a Dyad cannot be considered to be truly real since it exists only as a particular manifestation of the Nothing and quickly can return to nothing. This statement, although difficult to grasp with the modern brain, has been expressed in equally abstract modern concepts such as all of creation came forth from God who created the male and female, or creation came forth from *Brahmā* who created *Shiva* (male) and *Shakti* (female). The early *Vedas* described *Indra* who preceded *Agni* and *Soma* or Sun and Moon.

There is, of course, the generally accepted monistic philosophy of the Materialists which states that everything is physical with no spiritual counterpart. This philosophical view is atheistic and does not need refutation in this book.

There is another more integrative philosophical approach that considers that Nothing, as the Source by itself, is not real and only becomes real with the advent of the Dyad. Reality therefore must include both the Source and the Dyad. This approach using the Source and the two created elements can be called Trinitarian and is found in most religious descriptions of the manifesting of reality. In general, the "One" is expressed as the creative source or the ideation of the creation. The Sun (masculine force) is the process or energy of the bringing forth of the creation and the Moon (feminine force) is the manifested creation.

Any world that you find yourself in whether dream, real, past, future, parallel, or the self-created, has these three elements which define it or describe it. Most religions contain a Trinity encompassing these three elements which is symbolized within this book as the Golden Triangle.

For instance, Buddhism and Hinduism describe the world as having:

1. spiritual,
2. energizing, as well as
3. physical attributes.

The Christian Bible similarly describes the world as consisting of:

1. a Creator,
2. a manifesting Spirit, and
3. the manifested Creation.

The following text will use the three elements with the descriptions given in the *Parātriṃshikā* as:

1. the Creative,
2. the process of manifesting or *Mantra*, and
3. the manifested or *Mudrā*.

PART A

THE MOON OR THE PHYSICAL REALM

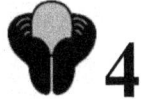

4

BONDAGE

"Become free from the conditioned Self
so that the inner power may rule."

Bhagavad Gita

"Truth shall make you free."

Universal

Sin: from Greek word *hamartana,*
meaning "to miss the prize or to err."

Bondage is a universal religious and philosophical term and it is used therein to mean enslavement to your own past. Bondage is normally tied to sin that has the universal religious connotation of being that which keeps you from reaching the rewards of life or the realization of your own dedications. A very important consideration is that what might be a sin to you such as lust may be a blessing and a positive force to a growing child, as will be discussed in Chapter Seven.

For almost all people in all cultures, social laws must be first learned and then obeyed. Citizens are therefore put into bondage of law. These laws are necessary for the growth of the children of that culture and hence cannot be labeled as sins. However, can the law become a sin to an individual who has followed and mastered the law? In other words, can the law keep an individual from further rewards of life? Does following the law lead to the ultimate or only reward in life? These questions are debated within many religions and can be bypassed for the moment with yet another question, "Is there anything higher than society and its law?" This last question is the basis for this first section of this book. In seeking the answer, the old story of Adam and Eve will be considered.

The story of the Garden of Eden is like many ancient religious stories in that there are generally two levels of understanding. The first level corresponds to the politically correct teachings of the time. The second level is called a hidden teaching open only to those who have attained a certain level of evolution. As you read the following version of the famous story watch your own reactions and look for problems that hinder you from following the narrative as an indication of your own bondage.

In the second level or rendition of the Garden of Eden, the heroes or good guys will be the serpent and Eve. This is in contrast with the normally accepted version in which they are the villains. As you read the story without the first and normal interpretation, another picture looms quite clear, that Adam and Eve are "pets" or watchdogs of the garden. The Bible states that they were created to "dress" and "keep" the garden. The original Hebrew words used to describe their position are: *abad* [pronounced "aw-bad" (dress)] that means to be enslaved in bondage, while *shâmar* [pronounced "shaw-mar" (keep)] is to guard.

Apparently, the gods felt that this particular pair of animals out of all of the different other types that they created might make good watchdogs. They were given all that they needed in terms of necessary food, shelter, etc. and all they had to do in turn was to be the watchdogs. The other central character in this scenario is the serpent. The Hebrew word for this serpent comes from *nachash* (pronounced "naw-cash") which means "to hiss" as whispering a magical incantation. The serpent was symbolic in most of the world for rebirth since it would crawl out of its old skin and grow a new one. As will be discussed later, the *Tantrik* system describes a "serpent" that lives in your sexual region and is capable of waking you and teaching you as does the serpent in this story.

As the hidden story unfolds, it becomes obvious that Eve is terrible as a watchdog. The essence of her "sin" is that instead of running a serpent out of the garden as instructed, she converses with it and befriends it. Who wants to keep a pair of watchdogs who not only let intruders in, but also befriend them? So of course, the gods ultimately kicked this pair out of the garden, and we can only assume that they then tried to breed a better pair.

Now the serpent was, in fact, wiser than the gods and could see the potential in this pair of animals. In fact, it could see that this pair of humans had more promise than any of the other animals that the gods had created and perhaps even more than the gods themselves. Therefore, the serpent told Eve of a source of knowledge that could offer her and her mate the possibility of ultimately becoming as great as or even greater than the gods by eating the fruit of the tree of good and evil. Of course, this possibility included hard work, pain, frustration, and challenges as well as joy. To get started on this path she had to sacrifice her security and tranquility, as well as her insipid and insentient life.

The attainment of knowledge opened her eyes to her own bondage and offered freedom from the confinement in the garden or kennel. This freedom shifted the responsibility for her life from the gods to herself. She chose to listen to the serpent, to eat of the fruit, and then to coerce Adam also to eat of it. This ability to guide and influence Adam also justifies her name as "life giver." Modern women are endowed with the potential of this "life giving" power, called *adhisthāna* in *Tantrik* writings, but generally are unaware of it and do not use it due to their conditioned roles in society.

To return to an overview of this story, the first level of interpretation is generally used with children giving the teaching that if you do not obey the laws, you may be punished with banishment. To a child could there be any greater punishment than to be banned from the security of his family? This version also teaches how other people may attempt to mislead you and cause you to lose all that you have. What parent is against this teaching? The main theme of the Garden of Eden is how wonderful it is and how you should appreciate it and do whatever is necessary to stay there. If this is transferred to loving and honoring your home, then this becomes a very positive teaching indeed.

Does this first level of interpretation, however, apply to adults as well as children? Are there not a majority of adults who cling tightly to security and refuse to open their worlds to other ideas, concepts, or teachings? They may very well defend their cherished ideas with their lives hoping for a future reward for their valor and view people with other viewpoints as threatening. To these people, the first interpretation is a panacea and an encouragement to try harder.

To discuss the second meaning of the story requires a great deal more effort. It must start with an understanding of bondage. Bondage is absolutely necessary if societies or social institutions are to remain stable. The members of any social group must conform to relevant requirements of skills, conduct, and purpose. The power and rights of a stable society must always be greater than those of an individual, and individual rights are well defined within the interests of that society. As an example, can you imagine driving down a high-speed freeway at 60 miles per hour with oncoming traffic without everyone observing the law? How long would your electrical power remain on if there were no laws concerning who ran the plants or maintained the machinery?

Bondage starts with social conditioning performed by families, churches, schools, and governments. As a child you were taught to follow laws beginning at a very early age with "potty" training during which you had to give up the control of your bowel movements to a higher authority. This was followed with the further suppression of basic instinctual impulses such as your hunger drive that was modified by table manners. Your language was impressed upon you along with a sense of values and definitions. Your basic fears were replaced with forced beliefs, inquisitiveness was replaced with fear of failure, and your sensual nature was replaced with shame about parts of your body. Perhaps the most surprising aspect of this process was the loss of feeling sensual or just physically good as the body was disciplined to become socially acceptable.

This early training or conditioning is not sufficient since there must also be a constant reminder or corrective force if a child veers away from the proper conduct. Societies utilize body language to enforce proper behavior and children are taught to become very much aware of it. For instance, a frown from someone instantly sets up tension within the child and the brain quickly reviews the current behavior with judgments as to acceptability. A parent will speak of how well their child behaves if they can control the child with just an approving or disapproving look.

A growing child is perceived by social institutions in terms of some future role in society. The child's conduct, manners, skills, and personality are then shaped to approach the idealized model of that future person. During this process, children are taught to be "true" to that role. The idealized person will have the traits of the teaching institution. For instance, a Catholic Church will tend to produce a person with Catholic beliefs, a farm family tends to produce farmers, and professionals raise teachers, doctors, lawyers, etc. The spoken language, gestures, dress habits, manners, and religious and moralistic views are all impressed into a child by social institutions during early formative years.

A subtle balance in behavior is maintained within a culture by the maintenance of two opposing forces controlling individual conduct. The opposing forces are recognized as "shoulds" conflicting with "should nots." For example, you should not be disrespectful to another person, but also you should not lie; you should not drive fast, but should not be late;

you should think kind thoughts, but you should protect yourself from harm. For almost every "should" there is an opposing "should not." The "shoulds" and "should nots" can be compared with the expansive and contractive forces discussed in Chapter Seven.

Self-control is therefore built upon pure frustration; you can never reach "perfection" since your conditioning prevents it. For instance, you want to succeed, but you should not be greater or better than those around you or else some calamity will happen. Similarly, you cannot fail so you flounder in between being a failure and a success. The controlling process ranges from uncomfortable to painful as we attempt to satisfy both the "shoulds" and the "should nots." The attempt results in maintaining a relatively unstable middle ground that provides the appearance of being in control. Experts in manipulating people are aware of this instability and can deliberately force the mind into one emotion after another until you become uncontrolled and unable to manage the large swing of emotions. The manipulator can thus gain control.

As an example, if a speaker adds a joke in the middle of a serious speech, the response of the audience will be far greater than if the joke were told in a normal social environment. If this joke is then followed with a statement that arouses fear, the fear will be far more intense than the humor. An experienced speaker can therefore sway the audience by controlling the sequencing of emotions while continuing to increase the intensity of them until the desired emotion or feelings are obtained.

The modern way of life is one of control and tension in which you attempt to present a rigid and fixed image of yourself to the outer world and to hide your real Self from scrutiny. The image to be presented is largely determined by television commercials and popular programs that present the "perfect bodies" or at least those that are in current vogue. Tummies are pulled in and the buttocks are tucked under, the shoulders are relaxed and eased forward while the head and neck are projected forward. You speak in a certain manner and what you say must likewise be currently acceptable, and what is even more frightening is that even what you think or feel must be subject to social acceptance. You are aware of a definite image of what you want to be and that image is made real. It is the reality and rigidity of the Self that proves the power of all of the social conditioning.

Once you take on a persona of being what you think you should be, it becomes hardened in place by your family and associates. If you fail to respond in accordance with your role, the people around you will let you know that you are not being yourself or inquire into what is wrong with you. As an example, if you forget to comb your hair, or speak from a different political viewpoint, your friends will quickly bring it to your attention. This is part of the problem visiting your parents because they expect you to behave and respond like you did as a child.

One of the higher powers cited by *Yoga* is the power of discrimination and this is required to fully ascertain the forces that have you in bondage. The early Christians called it "proving all things." Unfortunately, in our modern culture you are taught to believe rather than to prove or think and institutions take advantage of this serious lack in your development. As an example of how this lack of discrimination is used to put you further into bondage, consider the medical profession. This well-organized group uses fear to persuade large numbers of people to buy services offered by government or insurance-supported programs that guarantee health protection.

As an example, at the moment, breast cancer is being used to sell breast cancer clinics, research programs, and even more publications. The scandal starts with the statement that one in nine women will develop breast cancer. In order to obtain bondage to these programs, the news media add more fear and presently imply that one in nine women will die of cancer, but getting an examination will save your life. With a bit of discrimination, the actual death rate per year from breast cancer is less than 0.05%, whereas one in nine is over 11%. A bit of digging into the government statistics shows an even more revealing picture of medicine as indicated in Appendix B.

The figures all demonstrate that advances in modern medicine, including the introduction of the miracle drugs and intense cancer therapies, fail to show any increase in longevity. (The increase in deaths around 1920 shown in Figure 2 was due to a flu epidemic.) If modern medicine did in fact cure major diseases, then there should be a fast drop in death rates starting in the middle 1940's, yet no deviation in any of the curves can be noted. There is no significant difference between people who buy all of the health benefits they can, and Christian Scientists or people in Third World countries who use very little medicine if any. There simply is no evidence that medicine causes you to live longer.

However, products of the Western technology, such as the common window screen, modern sanitation as well as an improved diet, can be related to an increase in life expectancy for infants and children. Surprisingly, this does not hold for senior citizens who still live about the same allotted years as their forefathers.[3] The death rate from cancer is increasing slightly each year and for breast cancer this can be attributed to a number of possible non-medical reasons. The most obvious reason is that there is a higher percentage of women who are living longer (cancer is primarily a problem of old age). Also, some less often considered reasons are the restriction of breast movement and reduced stimulation.

One of the most insidious aspects of social bondage is the conditioning that you are not in bondage! The majority of people and for the majority of the time believe that they control their own lives, thoughts, and actions. The Book of Thomas gives an excellent test for how much control you have when it suggests that if you cannot take off your clothes and stand on them (in public), you are in bondage. To most people this test is impossible because of their conditioned view of themselves and of others. As you look more deeply into your behavior, the dominance of past learning or past programming (to use a computer concept) becomes evident. You are not completely free to do as you wish, and this becomes even more disturbing as you realize that your wishes are also programmed.

There are two major methods of breaking free from bondage to the body or conditioning. Both of these methods are primarily centered upon the senses of the body. The first is the path of asceticism wherein you break free of conditioned responses by diminishing your desires through the denial of any pleasures and the adherence to a totally enveloping law of conduct. The second is to increase the senses such that you look for more pleasure, trusting in a guidance or law beyond society and your own conditioned desires and thoughts.

The two paths of following religious law or seeking a higher law were debated by the early members of Christian groups, particularly since many of the early members were Jewish with a heavy tradition of obedience to the law. The path of law adherence and social obedience must be viewed as a necessary beginning path (for almost everyone) as the Self is developed and prepared for evolution. As Saint Paul in the Bible teaches, there are two laws, the lower and the higher. The lower path is followed in the

---

[3] See Appendix B, Figure 3.

first stages of evolution requiring judgment and control. The succeeding path of liberation is trodden by renouncing judgment and attachment to results as will be discussed in Chapter Seven.

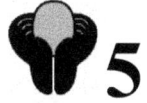

THE DANCE OF LIFE, *LĪLĀ*

Y ou sit beside a stranger, a person you have not met before nor will ever meet again. You are bored and feel isolated and have a deep yearning to find some relationship or union with someone. You become interested in the stranger next to you and wonder what she is thinking or feeling and find a desire to feel some interaction with her. You offer some simple statement and then…two hours later you part with a sense of deep union and sharing of extreme intimate feelings approaching ecstasy. There were no conflicts, only deep yearning and the sense of having been overpowered.

Why can you not have this closeness with your friends and family? The difference in the two states of interaction with the stranger and with your friends can be described as the difference between trusting what is happening or what is going to happen versus attempting to control the outcome by thinking and trying. This is the difference between freedom and bondage or "playing" and "trying." This difference will be elaborated upon in the next chapter.

Playing is first experienced as a child. Initially, a child may watch older children playing some imaginative interactive game. Then the child is gradually allowed to enter into the game, starting as an inert nonreactive element, like a crew member in a space game or a student in a school game. At this level the child is told what and when to speak and is fully controlled by the older children in the game. The child gradually senses the intensity the older children bring to the game and how they fully interact with each other, somehow not worrying or hesitating about what they do or say. The child senses magic in the game that overtakes and controls the players. In the game the children are able to let the game and their different roles dictate their actions, what they think, say, and do. Newcomers are gradually led into the method of game playing until finally the game controls their actions as well. When the game and not the older children control, then the child becomes a full-fledged player.

Educators and other people working with children are aware of the power of games. If a teaching or lesson can be inserted into a game, then

29

it is more rapidly absorbed by the children than if they "try" to learn the content.

What is of importance in these games is the ability of the children to accept various roles and to make them real in their own minds and perhaps even more importantly, to make them real in the minds of the other players. Once they assume and enliven their respective roles, they no longer have to think or plan "how" to play their roles in the game. They must, of course, continue to put their effort into maintaining the roles. The roles fit the game and the game seems to fit all of the roles. The game moves along with the children becoming more and more enmeshed within and taken over so that observing adults can become concerned about their children's fantasies becoming real, which of course they are. To play these imaginary games requires that the children have an initial dedication to the game or a deep yearning to become someone different, a willingness to renounce who they were before the game, and a trust in the game to guide them. The children must likewise be willing to let the game overpower them and control their thoughts, actions, and statements. This process is called *samarpana*.

Game playing is nearly opposite to the conditioned interaction with others that children eventually learn. In game playing, the role is of greatest concern. Effort must be placed into portraying the role just right. Even slight deviations of the role can ruin the game as for instance, smiling if you are playing a suffering dying martyr. The other point of interest is that in game playing there cannot be any effort put into what you are going to say or do. Instead, you must be completely open to the game and let the game lead you. In the adult civilized world, the concerns are reversed. You must worry about what you are going to say and do. At this time, you do not put effort into the role since that is assumed to be fixed and is the real "me."

Children are being civilized or conditioned to have fixed and controlled responses to the outside world, or to say and do prescribed things. Their role, ego, conditioned self, or character then becomes the result of doing the prescribed things in a prescribed way. This is of course the opposite to game playing.

The first game that a child learns to play is reacting to a parent. A child, for instance, will increase the intensity of a scream if it seems to yield more response from a parent. When children scrape their knees, they may look to a parent's response to gauge how much effort they should put into playing the role of an injured person. The parent becomes the leader or power behind each moment in the game. Later, this variable reaction to the parent becomes fixed, based upon success in the past. The response becomes a part of the conditioned self or ego.

Children are gradually taught by the adult society to be only one person or to have only one role (with fixed and repeatable responses to the outer world). This is evidenced by some of the definitions you have about someone, such as; they take everything seriously and frown, or they laugh at problems, or they are honest. While a child is being conditioned to maintain a fixed response to the world, they are also warned about people who are "playing" a role which might be misleading and harmful, such as a child molester who smiles and offers candy. This conditioning carries on into adulthood with adults being very suspicious of people "who are not themselves" including yourself. Just what the term "being your self" means is not questioned. The actor Peter Sellers was quoted as saying that he had played so many different roles that he no longer knew who he was.

The conditioned and rigid social reaction of adults requires many years of coaching, copying, and watching. When adults become parents, they find themselves rearing their children as they were reared. One of the humorous sides of parenting is the recognition that you are doing to your own children what you rebelled against in your parents. The professional games played out in the marketplace require studying, practice sessions, and much coaching.

College students learn more than coursework as they observe the mannerisms of their professors and later adopt many of them as their own. A person entering the blue-collar workplace also finds coaching and training from other workers in how to please the bosses, how to get along with fellow workers, and how to minimize the effort or pain in the work. The advent of unions and professional standards has complicated the drama and roles in the workplace, and the games are played with increasing sophistication.

When you consciously choose a game and play it with the understanding that a mystical unseen power in that chosen game controls the actions of the players, the game becomes "the dance of life." This dance of life requires dedication, renunciation, energy, and trust. You must fully intend to interact with the dance and do, say, or feel whatever the dance

31

requires. The role that you intentionally put on to play is called your *mudrā*. If you do not consciously choose a role or a game to play then you remain a conditioned robot with conditioned responses that are associated with "you."

The dance of life that includes others must therefore start with a clear agreement of the roles each active person involved in the game will play. If one person is playing the role of a policeman, then there must be the recognition of the power that goes with that role. The policeman role must have the power to control and to overpower you if necessary. A teacher role must be a perfect source of wisdom without flaw who can overpower you with new insights. A lover must have complete control over your feelings and be able to lead you into ever deeper intimacies. A physician must have mystical powers of healing which can overpower your illnesses or complaints. One of the very interesting aspects of the game of life is that when you empower the other players, they play their roles with greater intensities. As an example, if you do not empower your policemen, and instead consider them as part of your problems then they become ineffective in controlling. Similarly, when you limit the power of your lover, love and intimacy disappear only to be replaced with conditioned responses.

Your own role requires the acceptance of purpose and power and the renunciation of any old role that may have been played, including "being your self." You must have a clear concept of the goal associated with the role and its relationship to the chosen game, and then you must take on the attributes or characteristics that make that role and game become more and more intense.

If you are playing "being your self" for instance, then the goal is carried in your conditioning and may appear as "being good." The characteristics of the Self then take on the nature of being affable, agreeable, trustworthy, and traits learned from our childhood as being socially acceptable. If, however, you take on the role of being a fireman, for instance, then many of the old learned traits must be shed. Concern for Self must be replaced with concern for others. Fear of fire, height, or danger must be overcome with absolute trust in equipment, procedures, leadership, and fellow firemen.

Primitives living close to nature do not outgrow this trusting game and instead perceive the world as a unity and their immediate God as a Spirit contained or moving in everything (each element having its own nature, game or god). Nothing in nature acts upon its own, but rather as an interaction with everything else. If you attempt to live in nature without playing this game, you remain always an outsider and at harm. You may also argue a similar game in a city with its inhabitants becoming "street-wise" or acquiring other civilized games such as sales or construction.

One major source of misery to adults is the loss of the concept of playing a game. Instead, you start to identify with your role and see yourself as being that role, not a player acting that role. It is this identification with the role that immediately limits your ability to change or to evolve beyond the role. In contrast, you can accept the concept that what you think you are is only a role that you have been playing most of your life. This role was not of your choosing, but rather was forced upon you during the process of becoming civilized.

Public performers and artists report how some of them become identified with their role on stage and have difficulty in shedding it off-stage. "Groupies" or their followers increase the difficulty since they force the performer to continue their stage role off-stage. This is not unlike what happens when you, as an adult, are in the company of your parents and are forced into old roles.

The comparison between conditioned roles and the desired new roles is like the difference between reliance on past conditioning and shaping a new role that lies in the future. That desired role is ahead of the present moment in time, always in the future. As an example, when you are your old self, you "think" about what you should do, whereas in a desired role, you find yourself doing without thought. "Thinking" is the link with the past conditioning whereas "finding yourself," is reacting to that which is ahead in the unfolding or on-coming moment.

One interesting aspect of the game of life is that it cannot have a beginning or an ending. We must step fully into a role immediately upon entering it. You cannot gradually become a boss with an employee or gradually become a parent with a child. It is similar to dreaming. You enter a dream without any preamble and never have to ask, "What's going on?" or "Where am I?" You are instantly in a role that has a history as well as a present and future all controlled by the game.

The dance or game of life has no ending. If you encounter an old school friend after many years of absence, there is an immediate reconnection to the old game that you played together. Class reunions are interesting in that even after decades, the old school roles and interactions predominate despite what each individual may have done in the intervening years. There is a definite sense of continuing worlds with no time in between the scenes. You do not experience a time lapse between meetings with people who have been joined in play. By extrapolation of this experience, you see the impermanence of death or the ability of some inner spiritual nature to exist beyond physical separation.

The game of life cannot be coupled with the normal controlled world. You cannot enter into the game while attempting to restrain or control your actions or thoughts. It is an all or nothing type of interaction. Children, for instance, cannot play "mud slide" if they are concerned about keeping their clothes clean. Nor can you experience the joy of the game with a fellow traveler in conversation if you are concerned about saying something wrong. There must be a complete renunciation of other roles in order to play a new role even though the new role may have some characteristics that are similar to the old role.

In the marketplace, if you can renounce the desire to judge and control, you can learn to experience the game of life with people you would not normally choose as playmates. This stepping into the game of life can be accomplished even though those around your do not see the game. You may have opponents in the business world for instance, whom you have disliked very much, but this dislike may be changed to a respect for their abilities in playing their roles (even though they might deny that they are "playing").

If you can see your enemies as supporting players in the game of life, then they can be accepted as wonderful additions to the plot who increase the intensity of the game by their excellent portrayals of an opposing force. You learn to react to an individual's role with intensity while seeing the interaction as part of the whole play and loving the person playing the hateful role. This can be compared to a children's game where one child plays the role of some horrible fiend, hated by all but at the same time completely enjoyed by the other players. It is again when one identifies either the conditioned self or other individuals with the roles that misery results.

The game of life has the characteristic of "pulling" you into it. As you step into the game, the desire to act or react grows. The game intensifies and the game tends to find a rising crescendo as the players warm to it and develop skills that increase their ability to project their roles. The villain becomes more villainous while the heroes become more heroic. The game is fired by the desire to experience more and more in the game. This intensification of the action will be called the crescendo of the game or *vimarsha*. This crescendo, *vimarsha*, is well known to playwrights and musicians and reflects the intention of playing the game or listening to some music whereby you wish to be stimulated and carried beyond your present feelings.

For example, in the conversation described at the beginning of this chapter when you are bored with your trip and looking for a lively discussion with a fellow traveler, you allow a discussion to intensify and become more and more personal or intimate to increase the crescendo or interest in the conversation. If you are successful, the time passes almost instantly and you arrive at your destination actually refreshed and more alive than when you started the trip.

Unfortunately, as the excitement and crescendo increase, most would-be players may back away from the game and begin to judge their actions or feelings. They may then become horrified at their lack of self-control, the exposure of their inner feelings, or the animation in their expression. It is typical to start to feel that you are being overpowered by the other person or the game or both. Such an interruption destroys the game by removing the intimacy and the crescendo of the game. The game is reduced to a controlled social interaction.

To continue in the game, you must allow the *vimarsha* of the game to become overpowering and trust in the outcome. Along with the trust, there likewise is a requirement for a greater and greater input of energy (in a form that will be discussed later). As The game intensifies, you find that you are exerting yourself more and more with increased awareness and openness as well as with the intensity of your expressions. Without this increased investment, the game dies.

Another requirement is that you must not attempt to bring another world or game within the present game. For instance, one of the reasons that you can find a game with a stranger on a bus is that you can renounce your old games that include self-importance, prestige, social powers, etc. If you attempt to bring one of your old roles into this new game, the game will probably die unless the other person can build upon your old game.

In general, our conditioning labels activities with a *vimarsha* as "fun" or as "games" while the activities without a crescendo are the drudgeries of life. The method for increasing the joy in living is therefore to bring *vimarsha* into your ordinary activities or to make a game of each element of life.

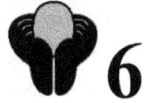

6

HEAVEN

"The kingdom of Heaven is within you...
unto everyone which hath shall be given; and from him that hath not,
even that he hath shall be taken away from him."

The Bible

The term "Heaven" was introduced in Chapter Three as the source of a creation and this chapter will add to that definition several more considerations including the idea that it is also the state of existence. Heaven, or the state of Heaven, has been commonly defined as a perfected world, but this is not a sufficient definition since it also becomes the source of creation of yet another higher world and hence cannot be perfect. Existence in a Heaven requires *vimarsha* or the seeking of more and more in your immediate experiencing of life. Heaven has some characteristics opposite to many of the common descriptions of Hell, such as eternal torment, unending suffering, and eternal bondage, but the common definitions of Heaven as a future place of eternal rest or peace lack *vimarsha* and become something like eternal sitting, which is not very appealing even if the sitting is done in a beautiful hall.

Heaven, as used in the ancient world, was not a place, a state of mind, or even something that could be directly described since it cannot ever be static. Jesus, in the Bible, gives excellent allegorical definitions of Heaven such that it is like ten virgins, a mustard seed, an inheritance that must be used, a pearl of great price, etc. When the ancient teachings are understood, then they provide the key to understanding these models as will be demonstrated. The following text will attempt to describe a few of the attributes of Heaven. As you read, do not attempt to form a complete or understandable picture of Heaven for it can only be understood during its creation.

To summarize Chapter Three, Heaven must come forth from a world that was created using the power of the Sun and Moon of a higher Heaven. The created world can in turn create another Heaven since that world must also contain the elements of creation, the Sun and Moon. This concept is

37

important in understanding the following text and for changing your own world into a Heaven.

You have probably experienced Heaven to some degree and you might have even stated that you were in Heaven. As for instance, when you have been caught up in the dance of life and lost your ego, judgements, and self-importance, you found a complete oneness with your inner mentally created view of what the outer world should be and what you perceived it to be. Your outer world became a perfect reflection of your own mind or creative center; or the inner Heaven became the source of the created perfect outer world. You may have done superhuman things or at least heard of others who have done so in this Heaven.

The above biblical phrase "Heaven is within you" is used for an introduction to this chapter because when it is interpreted correctly it shows the universality of the early concepts of reality. The original Greek word used for "within" (*en*) is not the specific Greek word meaning "inside" (or in the future), but rather has the sense of an intermediate position as between a source or creation and its full or final manifestation. This definition is strange to a modern Westerner and meaningless without more of the ancient concepts of reality. With this interpretation, however, the above statement about Heaven is in agreement with other ancient writings and can be understood to mean that you can be an integral part of Heaven in the present moment. This then leads directly to the opening question of the *Parātriṃshikā* which asks "How can you find this Heaven?"

Consider first a sequence of Heavens. The ultimate Creator of all is called the "One" in *The Emerald Tablet* and this "One" must reside in a creative Heaven that is called the Telestial Heaven. Out of the Telestial Heaven came the Sun and the Moon which reside in the Celestial Heaven and together are a manifesting of the "One." The "One" in the Celestial Heaven, or the Sun and Moon in turn created Earth which in its perfected form is called the Terrestrial Heaven or Heaven on Earth. This perfected Earth must involve you as a co-creator as will be discussed and requires a reflection of your inner perfection. This inner reflection is formed in part by your past experiences as well as your genetic inheritances or *samskāras*. When your dedication and yearning can be energized with the proper energy and *samskāras*, then Earth can become the kingdom of Heaven, *Anuttara* or state of perfection, *moksha* or freedom, enlightenment, etc.

Heaven is never the ultimate fulfillment, rather it is something always ahead of you. What is ahead of you is created with the mind or the power of the Masculine or Sun as will be discussed in *Part B*. To create Heaven, the conditioned "you" must become a co-creator with the inner Sun and Moon. You are, however, a creation or reflection of the Celestial Sun and Moon dyad and cannot be separated from it as discussed in Chapter Three, so therefore you also contain the Sun and Moon within yourself and hence are not only a co-creator, but also the creator.

This bit of logic sounds strange but is paramount to finding your personal Heaven. This identity with the higher realms will be dealt with in *Part B* of the book, but for the moment a reflection of the basic teachings of some of the religions can make this point somewhat clearer. You have basic building blocks within yourself described as: *Yin* and *Yang*, *Shiva* and *Shakti*, subtle and gross, Spirit and flesh, or Sun and Moon. Religions express these inner building blocks identically with those of the Celestial Heaven. If there is God in Heaven, the same God is within you. What is above, must also be below. What is without, must also be within.

This realization of the creation of Heavens immediately changes the approach to changing your life and world since the change must come from a Heaven above or beyond the Heaven you are attempting to create or enjoy. In other words, if you are not enjoying your world and want to change it, you must first find the Heaven or power that created it. This Heaven or power is beyond your present identification with the conditioned self who is in the midst of the world judging, desiring, and fearing. Most old religious writings attempt to teach this view by arguing that the physical and manifest world was first a mental creation in the mind of the "One" or Creator. The Bible, for example, has two creations in the book of Genesis; the spiritual creation (*mantra*) which existed before anything was made manifest and then the physical creation (*mudrā*) which became the manifest.

If you are not in the kingdom of Heaven, where are you then? In describing the normal world, you do not use the word "perfect" to describe it. There is a large difference between your expectations and desires for the outer world and what you observe. This can be expressed as a large difference between your inner *mantra* and your projected *mudrā*. This difference can be explained with the model of a child's world. If a child is lost in play, then there is complete agreement between the inner world of the child and the outer world. The game has become the perfect reflection of the inner mind or *mantra*. When the child, however, enters into the world controlled by adults, there is suffering because of the vast gulf which separates the outer world from that created within. Further, social institutions desire to keep the gulf in place to maintain conformance.

The conditioned world of the adults and society can be called the "World of Law" or that of Mammon, while the higher and opposing world can be called the "Kingdom of Heaven." The two realities or worlds can be described with four basic elements such as:

Heaven

1. You must maintain the dedicated game and role you have chosen.
2. You cannot worry or attempt to control any thoughts, actions, or feelings.
3. There must be a continual crescendo of feelings or *vimarsha* in your world as you surrender to the role.
4. There must be an intense faith in the game and its outcome.

World of Law

1. The role is fixed as being "yourself."
2. You must be proper and do that which is expected by controlling what you say and do.
3. You do not allow yourself to become overpowered or to increase the intensity of life or *vimarsha*.
4. You maintain a tight control on your thoughts and actions through continual judgements.

It is true that you are either in Heaven or in the World of Law. You cannot be partially in the kingdom of Heaven. There are, however, some people who may be said to be preparing to enter Heaven or are finding moments during which they are caught up in it. It is the study of these people that became the basis for *Yoga* and more recently became the basis of study for the American psychologist, Abraham Maslow.

Maslow studied highly evolved or exceptionally successful people and is credited with being the founder of the Humanistic Psychology movement. In studying the exceptional people of society (as did the ancient sages), rather than those of lesser social attainment, Maslow found that the exceptional or "self-actualized" people had characteristics that can be related to the special traits associated with religious or spiritual mastery. Maslow suggested six steps required to reach this higher state of attainment. These compare quite closely with the Eastern concepts of the steps necessary for evolution as discussed in the next chapter. Many of the modern Humanistic movement members have, however, concentrated on the lower steps in Maslow's "hierarchy of needs," which are the beginning social conditionings of people, rather than on the higher steps of evolution. This exclusion is obvious since Maslow pointed out that less than 1% of a populace reaches the higher realm. This is an interesting number when compared to the statement in the Gospel of Thomas that only one in a thousand reach the state of Heaven. Does this mean that only one in ten of Maslow's self-actualized people reach the kingdom of Heaven or has the world evolved since Thomas' day?

One characteristic that impressed Maslow was that the self-actualized have a humility and openness rather than having a rigid self-centered view of their world. Along with this humility is a deeper insight into the nature of the Self and outer world with an ability to be more objective and observant of life. They are able to "see" and "hear" truth, whereas the majority of people "hear" and "see" only that which they desire or are conditioned to hear and see. The self-actualized have broad interests and are capable of non-judgmental and correct interactions with their world.

One strong characteristic that all of the self-actualizing individuals have is an intense dedication or drive toward some major goal in life. Because their goal becomes central to their life, everything becomes pleasurable whether others perceive it as work or play. They are highly creative with their creativity "flowing through" similar to that found in children. They are uninhibited and can play almost any role demanded of them. Lastly, they have an abundance of courage and faith in their own future and capabilities. These characteristics can be perceived to be fundamental for being in the kingdom of Heaven as described in the Sermon on the Mount by Jesus.

Another often quoted characteristic of Heaven is having a particular state of love. This state of love is not "caring for," "controlling," "possessing," or in "pleasing" another person. Instead, the higher state of love can be expressed with the *Sanskrit* word *samaj*. There is no corresponding English word for *samaj*, though you have probably experienced it at some time in your life.

Samaj is described as having three powerful forces associated with it:

1. A yearning to merge with another.
2. The ability to completely surrender to another.
3. The opposing conflicts to the above two.

The first term of yearning is not a passive term but requires a continuous driving force for more union or for coming ever closer; it is not becoming accepting, comfortable, or accustomed to each other or fully understanding each other. In *samaj* as in Heaven there must forever be the reaching and yearning for more and more. Surprisingly, that state can be found and is a characteristic of Heaven. The first term is not the same as wanting to possess or please each other.

The second term of surrendering is foreign to most modern people as they attempt to control their own lives and prevent others from influencing them. This term means surrendering to the extent that your mind and body become overwhelmed or controlled by the other. You are thoroughly conditioned not to allow yourself to be influenced by anyone else, particularly your enemies or those you don't like. *Samaj*, however, requires you to reach into and join another person's beliefs, feelings, and thoughts as if they were your own. As an example, a wise person can often be characterized by his willingness to listen to any issue with an open mind, whereas you may have trouble listening to any statement in support of your opposite political party or religion. One further example of surrender is given by young children who are able to open to and learn opposing points of view and agree with both.

Before moving on to the third term, the interaction of the first two terms needs to be clarified. An excellent example of *samaj* is sometimes perceived in "first love" as two teenagers fall in love. They are said to exist in their own world and to hold each other in the palms of their hands. They desire nothing more than to merge with the other in complete union in body, mind, and soul and at the same time to allow the other to overpower them as they surrender to whatever the demand of the other might be. Whatever one says to the other is wonderful, true, and has a tremendous interest and power over the other. Parents can be very jealous of the power another person has over their child and to most people in the modern world, this love is foolish, irresponsible, and degrading.

At this stage of love the third term of conflict can start to be understood. It is perhaps the judgment of the lovers by others that begins the process of conflict between the two. The people surrounding this couple warn them about being overcome, how they cannot trust each other, why the love cannot last, and about the weaknesses of one or both of the lovers. Because of these comments and expressed doubts, the couple will typically try harder to prove their love and the lovers start to constrain or increase their actions, thoughts or statements, so as not to endanger the relationship. This trying, constraining, and proving changes the yearning and surrendering into pleasing the other and others and controlling the self to prevent any reduction in the relationship.

However, they are now relying upon their learned and programmed concepts of what "should be" rather than "what is."

Rather than "losing" themselves in their love, they now attempt to control their actions such that their love is not threatened. They can neither have an open, deep, and ever-increasing yearning, nor can they surrender and become completely overcome by the other because of the fear of losing what they once started to experience. All of the attempts to control become conflicts that prevent love. The above opening quotes from the book of Luke in the Bible can be seen to directly relate. When the lovers trusted the "kingdom of Love" that lay within themselves they found more and more riches, but when they lost their faith and attempted to preserve and keep what they had, they lost it.

A true union between two lovers can only take place with deep yearning and sacrifice of the self to the other. The higher plane relationships must be first experienced and then the relationship itself must be trusted which requires an unsubstantiated and unrelenting faith. Without this faith in their own potential future, the lovers are doomed to reducing their love. Their love can quickly drop to the possessive, jealous, and controlling relationship so familiar to almost everyone as they work at and cling desperately to what they were taught that they should have. Another important point about conflict is the element of giving you free Will. Without conflict, it would be impossible to escape *samaj*. This can be related to seeking Heaven, without opposition or conflicts you would have no free agency or choice and hence, you would be powerless and remain only a kept "pet."

Love, like the dance of life and ecstasy (that will be discussed in Chapter Twenty), must continually be increasing and have *vimarsha*. The excitement, enjoyment, or ecstasy of a relationship with someone else is dependent upon the rate of exploring or sharing new experiences with the other. The social relationships exist because of fixed and generally well-defined boundaries around each person. Social decency for instance, requires that you not stare or even react to a facial blemish on a casual acquaintance. Personal questions or even observations are taboo and inter-actions must be kept at an impersonal level.

This boundary, however, gradually lessens or opens with increased contact as you both gradually expose yourself more to the other. It is this increase in exposure that becomes pleasant or intriguing. In most social relationships, however, a stable boundary or separation develops which is "comfortable" to everyone. There is an unwritten list of taboo subjects that are avoided and limitations on behavior are recognized. For instance, any deviation in your opening remarks or your normal facial expressions on greeting these people causes an immediate negative or questioning response.

In an exciting relationship, on the other hand, participants find that with each encounter, the boundaries open more and more as they both learn more of the other and share more experiences. This opening can involve much pain as well as relief as deeper feelings and thoughts are shared. This opening of boundaries is enhanced with the common pursuit of some goal and in sharing the problems and successes of the past toward that goal. If the relationship does not include some mutual evolution, love or *samaj* becomes less as the shared boundaries become fixed, and the conflicts become hardened.

The parables of Jesus about the kingdom of Heaven are unique in religious writings. However, they are seldom elaborated upon because of the misleading way they are generally interpreted. The actual power in the parables about the kingdom of Heaven is that they express a universal experience that rises above the normal World of Law and may be unassociated with any religious belief or practice. As an example, and as an introduction to *Tantrik* philosophy, consider the Sermon on the Mount as described in the book of Matthew in the Bible.[4]

This Sermon is an ancient "technical" commentary in that the meaning of terms is developed step-by-step (*krama*) and each verse must be taken in sequence. The necessary state of mind is given in the opening Beatitudes by the usage of Greek terms which specify humbleness and openness and the ability to allow the outer world to overpower you similar to Maslow's observations. The teaching of the Sermon follows with a definition of the power within yourself as "the Father in Heaven" which must be compared to the indwelling masculine force (or Sun) popularly called *Shiva* in the earlier *Tantrik* writings. (*Shiva* is also considered to reside in the Celestial Heaven as well as within your body.)

It is this acceptance of an inner Masculine force that makes the rest of the Sermon understandable. Much of the following text points to the intense effort that it takes to stay in this Kingdom which can be compared to the difficulty children have in playing an imaginary game. The most challenging aspect of remaining in this state is that you must follow stricter laws than any religion can require.

The Sermon can be compared with the characteristics of the self-actualizers studied by Maslow such as humility, faith, openness, and trust. Jesus elaborated upon trusting the game of life with his statements of taking no thought for tomorrow, or for what you will say, do, or even wear which are, of course, contrary to religious requirements of constantly trying to be good.

In addition to the Sermon on the Mount, Jesus provided many different allegorical models to define the elusive concept of Heaven. The opening quotation from Luke above gives Jesus' concluding remarks on the parable of the talents. This parable depicts various people being given money (talents) and how the one who invested, used, and increased the money is praised while the others who carefully hid and secured their money had to give up what remained. The teaching of the parable of the talents is also reflected in the above story of the teenage lovers who in attempting to preserve their love, lost it.

---

[4] See Table 5, *Part E.*

Another parable of Jesus uses the model of the seed that contains all of the future manifestation of a life (as does *Tantra* in the game of life or *Līlā*). This can be seen in reviewing portions of your life when you dedicated yourself to some attainment and then found the unfolding of your world to the perfection of your dedication. It is as if there was a master plan or seed contained within your first dedication.

A third parable uses the idea of "leavening" as do many major religions. Leavening was associated with a spirit that changed the nature of ground grain or flour and was symbolic of the transformation of an individual infused with a higher spirit of life. The last two models can therefore be used to imply that the kingdom of Heaven is contained within yourself (like a seed) or that you must be infused with a Spirit which will permeate and flow throughout your entire being (like leavening) to thoroughly change your life. Jesus also likened leavening to activating the whole loaf or the entire game (in our parlance) which fits the requirement that a game must continually grow or contain *vimarsha*. Further, if you do not fully contribute to a game, to continue the analogy, you cannot remain a player as Jesus exemplified with the story of the ten virgins and their lamps.

The state of being in Heaven is being compared directly to the trust and dedication required to play a child's imaginary game as described in the last chapter. With trust the child dives into a role completely, becoming a character and gaining fully the powers associated with that character. Children will report how the power of a role can overpower them and lead them into a previously unknown experience. If they do not respond to this power, they remain outside the game, locked in the effort of controlling or judging themselves such as a child who is afraid to get his clothes dirty.

Another approach to the attainment of Heaven can be described using the Indian model of the four objects or stages of life. The four objects or stages of life with their four major goals are: *dharma*, or the obedience to the World of Law; *kāma*, or the seeking of joy; *artha*, or the reaching for wealth and power; and *moksha*, perfection or liberation. Each of these stages has an associated sexual nature that will be discussed in detail later. Each stage or object also has a Power or creative source attributed to it as well. A child begins under the power of the World of Law or the manifested and Terrestrial Heaven. Although the next major objective involves the desire for joy with associated power of the Moon, the child is taught to distrust joy and consequently, the power of the Moon. Later, when success is the major goal, involving the power of the Sun, the child is

46

taught to measure success only in terms of dollars, which likewise diminishes the power of the Sun.

Western institutions do not in general support the ancient four stages of life since they do not advocate the latter three objects of life and instead argue for devotion to duty and finding security and safety. The average life is a Triune of law, joy, and success, whereas the higher life becomes a Triune of joy, success, and perfection. The four stages and the associated sexual force with its source are listed on the next page.

Stage	**Duty** (*Dharma*)	**Joy** (*Kāma*)	**Success** (*Artha*)	**Perfection** (*Moksha*)
Sex	Neuter	Feminine	Masculine	Androgynous
Power	Terrestrial Heaven	"Moon"	"Sun"	kingdom of Heaven

Trusting in the higher power of a game or of Heaven conflicts with our modern Western culture in two major ways which prevent most people from "playing" or stepping into the kingdom of Heaven. The first problem is that the religious organizations require that game playing be postponed to a life after death and also that you must put your efforts and judgements into being good. This process leads, of course, into further conditioned control. The second problem is the belief in the powerlessness or nonexistence of a higher power ruling a game. You may have turned against the concept of a benevolent God sitting on a throne watching your every action. But in doing so, you have thrown out any acceptance of a higher power or the Divine over your life. This denial forces you to the belief that you must control and judge your own life according to your conditioned responses.

One further comment about the "power" of the Divine: The Divine must have infinite and unlimited power if you are to fully play the game. The power of the game you are currently playing must become greater than any conditioned power or concepts. For instance, many people say that they believe in God, but then limit the powers of that God by not accepting anything in their life that does not meet their requirements of what God can and cannot do! In a game, you expect to do the unexpected and the miraculous, but that can only come with unlimited faith in the game and yourself.

This can be compared with a child who is told to, "Go and play, but don't get dirty or forget to be good." A strong warning is required here: The kingdom in Heaven is in no way similar to "doing what you want to do." Rather, it involves losing your desires as you allow a dedication to become manifest through the process of *mantra*. All of the world's major religions, as well as the great contributors to society, state that the kingdom of Heaven (or its equivalent) is attained only with a strong drive toward some evolutionary goal.

One important aspect of Heaven is the realization of super-normal powers often associated with it. Maslow was very impressed with the abilities of the exceptional people in his study and how they exhibited insights and actions that were certainly beyond the normal. As noted earlier, children often demonstrate actions, insights, and awareness beyond their usual ability when completely absorbed in a game as do partners in early love. The old system of *Tantra* stated that super powers come when there is a need for them; so, a first requirement is that you find yourself in a place where super powers are required of you. If you find yourself playing (with all of your effort) the role of an advisor, you will find that your advice is beyond what you could have given outside of the game. If you find that you are suddenly required to perform some feet of strength or courage, you may later be amazed at the power that comes forth.

For instance, consider a commonly reported type of incident in which a small woman lifts a car to release a child pinned under it. Initially with the shock of seeing the child trapped, the woman experiences a distortion of time, awareness, and capability of response. With trauma induced clarity, she sees the situation in complete detail. Then within the same time frame, she envisions herself freeing the child. The woman then simultaneously steps into that perceived role lifting the car. This is an example of the instantaneous transport into the kingdom of Heaven which should convince everyone of the supernormal powers that can be found.

Therefore, under sufficient duress and with sufficient faith, a new Self is created instantly which is able to deal with the pressures and demands of the moment, whether it be increased patience, strength, endurance, knowledge, or love. An important aspect of this new state is that the conditioned judgmental aspect of the self is bypassed and you view the world dispassionately without judgment, fear, or need to control. Normally, however, this change is not permanent and can only exist as long as the extreme demand exists. Once the demand ceases, you return back to your conditioned lower world and self. The practices of *Tantra* as will be described allow this normally hidden kingdom of Heaven to be attained, sustained, and utilized under intentional control for increased evolution, joy, and ecstasy.

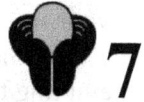

THE SEVEN MAJOR STAGES
OF EVOLUTION

Most of the world's religions originally taught that you have the chance of evolving upward step-by-step, from one level to another, from life to life, or from one world to another. As you look at history, an ever-increasing rate of evolution is obvious from generation to generation. Though most modern institutions teach that either chance or a Deity directed this evolution, the early writings state that the world evolves by the efforts of its inhabitants or that they at least share in it with an inner higher power. One important aspect of this book is demonstrating that individuals can and do evolve and are capable of creating new worlds and affecting the worlds to come.

Many of the world's great people report having changed their lives or to have stepped into new roles and worlds within their own lifetime. You also may have experienced stepping into strangely new worlds after puberty, marriage, trauma, or change in lifestyle. The ancients made a study of what happens as you enter into a new world and found that there are seven basic steps that have to be negotiated in mastering that world. The creation of worlds from a perfected Heaven and then the perfection of the new world into a new Heaven has been discussed in previous chapters. This chapter will discuss a particular aspect of this process, namely, the steps taken within each world leading toward its perfection or your own. (There is no difference between the two.)

Evolution is the mastering of a world or the accumulation of skills, powers, wisdom, and experiences that can then open you to a higher world for a repeat of the process. If this evolution is studied, a number of discrete steps can be described that are universal in any world. For instance, the word "wonderment" was used by a senior citizen stepping into a world called second childhood. This is the same sensation that is experienced in any major change in life such as marriage, deaths, professional appointments, moving, or any change that places you in a new position in terms of the people and/or places or the games around you. As you attempt to adapt to the new world, there is the development of frustration and anger

51

at your own ineptness that you typically will attempt to blame on someone or something else. As an example, it is common for many people attempting to step into a religious life to create or use a church concept of evil forces to blame for their inability to fully adapt to love, faith, or service.

Before proceeding on with the seven steps of evolution, the concept of good and evil needs further elaboration. The concept of good and evil forces or forces of light and darkness are institutional inventions. The older writings, on the other hand, speak of Light and Dark forces often as the Sun and Moon with both very much required for reality and evolution. This chapter will add another aspect to the Sun and Moon, namely the expansive nature of the Sun and the contractive nature of the Moon. The expansive force is called evolution or *pravritti* and the contractive force is called involution or *nivritti*.

Evolution and reality results from the expansion of your awareness outward and then the concentration (contraction) upon a very limited aspect of the total world such as a flying bird. As the world or your concentration is narrowed, the bird becomes real. Otherwise, the bird blends into the totality that is unreal or without specific form and definition. Similarly, you have a basic nature that you may call "goodness" which is essentially expansive as you open to the outer world. You also have a nature that is labeled bad as you turn inward with "emotions."

However, as will be discussed, the "emotions" serve to fuel or stimulate another reversal outward for more evolution. The following Table is presented as an overview of the steps used in evolving toward the kingdom of Heaven. Different cultures have used variations in the following listing, but the variations are unimportant if the basic concept is gained. The Table breaks the steps into three major divisions:

- the first is the growth and evolution within a social group or institution (the right-hand path),

- the second is the evolution as you choose your own path to be followed (the left-hand path), and

- the third is the opening into the kingdom of Heaven which will be discussed in detail later.

The numbered steps begin with a broad term of definition, followed by an evolutionary force, the corresponding contractive force, and finally the *Sanskrit* term for that step or level. The evolutionary force describes the inner Self expanding outward, and the contractive force, which is generally called a sin, is in actuality a necessary force in evolving. The last three levels describe breaking free of the World of Law and evolving toward perfection or the kingdom of Heaven and constitute "the left-hand path" of *Yoga*.

World of Law

Right-Hand Path	Emotion	Step/Level
1. Learning Basic Social Laws	Stillness Anger	*Vedāchāra*
2. Self-Control	Trust Envy	*Vaishnavachāra*
3. Self-Motivation	Chaos Lust	*Shaivachāra*
4. Developing	Discipline Pride	*Dakshinachāra*

The Higher Realm

Left-Hand Path	Emotion	Step/Level
5. Individualism	Vitality Sloth	*Vāmāchāra*
6. Perfected	Serving Avarice	*Siddhantachāra*

7. Freedom	Evolving Gluttony	*Kaulachāra*
Kingdom of Heaven		*Anuttara*

The above seven steps are again undertaken in a new world as you evolve through a sequence of worlds and Heavens.

The first level begins with your awareness of external forces. This is the beginning of evolution as the distinction between the inner and outer worlds is manifested. The inner stillness becomes the center for reaching toward the external. As you reach, you experience frustration and then anger as you discover the inability to bring the experiences and objects of the outer world into your center. Anger brings your awareness to a specific object and intensifies its relationship to you. This intensification makes it "real."

Learning control of the body, senses, and mind begins with success in interacting with the outer world as you desire to break through the separation of the inner "me" and the outer "it" interface. When you are a child, this interacting is generally assisted by a parent or sibling and they play with you encouraging you to reach, feel, and move. The joy of the interaction and experiences and the awareness that it can be repeated increase your trust in your own senses and body as well as the outer world. It is at this second stage that you, as a child, become trainable and can be conditioned to follow laws.

Self-control starts with the simple attempt to balance the expansive and contractive elements of reaching and experiencing. As your awareness of consequences is still very limited and the forces experienced in the outer world are constantly increasing, you find it expeditious to be guided by someone more experienced in worldly matters and trust in others begins. With trust, a model of behavior can be accepted and you can then attempt to comply with the new requirements of experiencing. Anger and frustration have been replaced with trust. With trust of the outer world, you also find envy. Others are perceived as doing incomprehensible things or enjoying things that cannot be directly understood. All of that appears to be wonderful and yet impossible to attain. You want it too.

The third stage of self-motivation results from the increasing force of envy and the desire to know and become more and more. You find that you have a power to reach out and that there is a corresponding reaction from the outer world that can be pleasant or unpleasant depending upon your judgements of the outer world. Pleasure is expansive in that your input and interest keeps increasing, whereas work is contractile as your efforts and awareness diminish. You find pleasure when you are "good" and are rewarded and you seek to obtain more pleasure. However, in seeking more pleasure or in being good, you encounter the chaos and uncertainty of the outer world and must constantly learn to judge with the Self as the center. That which results in unpleasant reactions must be renounced while that which results in pleasure is pursued.

In attempting to judge and equalize your world, you have the increasing awareness of unpredictability, lack of control, and of the unexpected that places you in a new state of chaos. You can no longer simply "be good" in an ever-changing world, but rather you are now required to exert yourself further by "doing good" or at least attempting the appearance of doing good before the outer world.

It is during the reaching for rewards and pleasure that lust develops. Those things that appear to have the highest pleasure become those things most lusted for. As lusts become unfulfilled, a new reaction occurs, a withdrawal from the outer world. The frustration that results when pleasure cannot be obtained now becomes unpleasant in itself.

This third level is reached by the majority of people in any society and is characterized by the ability to manage one's ambitions and desires to a level of controlled limitation. This involves reaching out to the extent that lusts and desires appear to be somewhat satisfied, but also contracting and withdrawing from interaction or involvement that requires too much effort or that may be judged negatively. It is the play of these two expansive and contractive forces that stabilize the members of a society much the same way that automatic controls work. For instance, a thermostat wants heat until a preset temperature is reached where it must turn heat off. Most people want success with a limited amount of effort, with the avoidance of notoriety or loss of privacy.

The fourth level requires increased effort and dedication. It is characterized by increased self-discipline with a goal of self-perfection or of doing good. A few people in a society have an inner drive to succeed which calls forth an expenditure of greater than average energy. They have a definite goal or dedication in their lives which they strive to attain. It may start with the desire to imitate some hero or heroine, a parent, or some fictional character, and the desire to take on the personal nature of that model "god" as much as possible. This effort immediately requires strong personal discipline as they learn, acquire skills, and develop a demeanor that radiates the personality of that personal god.

The expansive process of perfection is limited or modified by judgments leading either to delight in your progress or criticism of yourself at failure to reach expected goals. The delight can strengthen to the extent that it is judged by others to be pride, or similarly the criticism can lead to self-denigration. Either contractile force can become strong enough to stop further evolution, and many fail due to the inability to renounce either their pride or their self-denigration.

In order to renounce pride or self-denigration, another assessment of the self must take place. This perspective must become different from the limited social view of the self. Almost everyone is conditioned to view themselves within limitations of both potential success and failure. You are conditioned to stay within societal limits, neither too great nor too low in the eyes of the immediate milieu. It is at this level that you need to look beyond the expectations of conformance within the culture and define a higher goal or model for yourself. This model is the start of true individuality.

The fifth level begins the evolutionary steps toward the manifesting of your own Heaven called the stage of individualism. In attempting to break free from the confining and limiting bondage of the expectations and controls of society, another source of energy must be found that can be activated from within rather than from external sources. In order to stand alone and rise above the society, an independent, supportive, creative, and radiant force must be developed or found. This force results from the primal sexual energy that we will call *shakti* to be described later, and has as one of its attributes the shifting of the perceived outer world as it is called into usage. As we find the *shakti* to break free of conditioned judgments and their limitations, we find opportunities, challenges, and a beauty in the world, instead of drudgery and problems. This is the beginning of the higher world spoken of in religions.

There is a tendency initially to believe that you can throw out society and institutions and forget your past, but this misconception is quickly dispelled as you also become aware of the richness that your life has given you. You start to experience that the characteristics that you had labeled objectionable about yourself are in fact positive characteristics that have added to your richness. Instead of breaking free from your old teachings and concepts, you find that you build or stand upon them. Instead of driving down the highway on any side that you choose, you find yourself an even better driver as you increase the safety of yourself and others.

You are also able to directly recognize greatness in others and to see their true contributions to society. You are also starting to become one of the self-actualizers described by Maslow.

As you rise, you also become aware of the depths. With the ever-increasing effort and flow of *shakti*, you are at any moment, able to check your rise to success and reverse your direction toward inaction and oblivion. It is at this level that you are finally able to die spiritually. As long as you were a part of the lower world you could not separate yourself from yourself or separate the inner Sun and Moon as will be explained. Since at the lower levels you cannot separate yourself from your life, this gives rise to the Eastern concept of *samsara* or being bound to the wheel of continual birth and death. However, at the higher level where *shakti* is utilized, you can actually develop sufficient energy to remove yourself from the system of *samsara* by intentionally seeking ultimate death or oblivion.

The sixth level of evolution is called the stage of power or mastery. In facing oblivion, you can turn and see creation. In rising above the lower world, you can sense something which can survive your birth and death. Entropy can be reversed; you can leave behind something more than memories or ashes. Your life can produce a permanent change in the world contrary to the laws of physics. Your efforts and dedication, rather than being acts of uncovering or discovering, become the acts of creation. You are contributing to the creation of a new world and Self. Finding service to others is not in meeting their desires, but rather in planting seeds that can grow and change their very nature as they evolve. You become a creator in the kingdom of God. One very important aspect of "you" at this level, is that "you" become the tool for playing the higher game. "You" find yourself doing great works rather than "trying" to do good as a higher power takes over and controls your life.

As you look out over the unlimited domain, you can also look at your own shortcomings in the human form. The contractile forces make it easier to avoid looking at creating, and enjoy instead the possessing of all that is already created. Avarice is then fed with denial of our actual capabilities and possible future.

The seventh and last stage in your world is called the stage of freedom. Avarice can inspire the desire for even better worlds than those already existing. In denying your own abilities, you long for even greater powers. This sets in motion the creation or ascendancy to higher worlds and the evolution of your Self into more light and ecstasy. You become free of all of the limitations of the past worlds and instead become free to choose, select, create, or rule new worlds.

Before that moment of freedom, contractile forces can again make you reach for what is immediate. With the evolution you have undertaken, you can finally satisfy avarice to the extent that your whole world becomes the manifesting of that avarice. Avarice disappears in its own fulfillment. With its fulfillment, *vimarsha* and dedication also disappear. In gluttony you have gained mastery over worlds in order to create a complete world dominated by the object of gluttony. You can condemn yourself to perfected Hells of your own creation instead of finding freedom from the old.

The eighth stage is the first stage in another world or Heaven. As you free yourself from an old world and create a new world, that new world must likewise be explored and you must again evolve upward within it. This is the *samsara* of the East or the cycle of birth, death, and rebirth. This *samsara* can, however, always have the evolutionary aspect of finding more and more challenges, or more and more ecstasy in the direction of becoming a god or goddess.

8

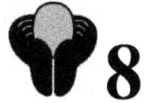

THE MYSTICAL NATURE OF
CHANGE

*"In the beginning
was unbounded energy and knowledge,
out of which came all that is."*

Physics

In attempting to describe the origin of the universe, modern science
generally assumes an initial pool of energy that then changes to become the physical universe that we now know. It is also necessary to
assume that a directive power commonly called "Physical Law" exists
behind this transformation of energy into space, time, and matter. This law
contains the knowledge as to what can and cannot take place and becomes
the master plan similar to that contained within the ancient mustard seed
analogy described earlier. Ever since the earliest days, science has been
consistently attempting to determine what the master plan or the knowledge of the universe may be.

Energy and Knowledge are not related or exchangeable. They are separate entities yet bound together in their mutual creations. They are the
ancient Moon and Sun or the Feminine and Masculine forces. The early
religions believed that within your sexual region lay a connection with the
Knowledge controlling the universe as well as a connection to the Energy
of the universe. You become god-like when you can utilize these two
forces to create new worlds or Heavens.

You are accustomed to change in the physical world, yet you must
become aware that any change, including becoming emotional, worried,
or having a thought, requires energy. To become aware and conscious of
that change also requires energy and then to deliberately and consciously
change your Self requires yet even more energy.

In the following discussion, an ancient concept of what energy is will
be added to what the modern world knows about energy. This can be done
since both ages agree as to the basic nature of energy, and while this

59

modern world pursued the energy of the industrial world, the ancients also pursued the energy of thought and inner transformation.

Both ages agree that energy is a mystical formless substance since energy cannot be directly measured, touched, weighed, or seen. Both the old wisdom and the new agree that energy can only be evidenced during some change. A stick of dynamite may weigh the same as a wooden stick, yet the actual differences can only be observed when the energy in both is released or changed into heat or an explosion. Similarly, a can of gasoline can be of the same volume as a can of water, yet the water can readily be determined to have far less energy than the gasoline when a match is brought near to them both. Observing the gasoline breaking into flame, the ancients would have stated that the gasoline contained a great deal of phlogiston, "fire element," or energy. In the modern world. science can measure how much "phlogiston" is in a can of gasoline by burning it and measuring the heat that results or they can calculate it from prior experiments with gasoline.

One of the chief problems with energy is that it can take so many different forms. It can appear in varied forms such as sound, motion, chemical, thermal, electricity, light, and life. There is a hierarchy within the various forms of energy based firstly upon the ability of a particular form to produce other forms of energy and secondly upon the concentration of that energy. As an example, this hierarchy can be seen in the production of electricity that can be used to produce many other forms of energy such as light and microwave radiation for cooking. Chemical energy in the form of coal is used to create heat and then the heat forms steam which drives a turbine that drives a generator that produces the electricity. Each step seemingly a higher form of energy, yet each step is essential in its proper order. The concept of a hierarchy and concentration of energy must be considered in causing change. Most of the members of the modern society recognize this in terms of their physical world as for instance, no one would consider using the sound from a radio to boil water. However, when it comes to changing thoughts, emotions, health, the perceived inner and outer world, as well as your creativity and interaction with others, ignorance and superstition prevail.

If a change occurs in life, there must be an expenditure of a discrete amount of energy. This is obvious in moving a piano up a flight of stairs, but not so obvious in changing one's mind although one might be aware of the mental struggle that preceded the change. You learned in school that it takes a particular type of energy to heat your house and to propel your automobile, but what and where is the energy to change your feelings, consciousness and thoughts and how do you find it and use it? Surprisingly, this is a question that modern scientists cannot fully answer even though they are able to measure and predict very well the flow and transfer of energy in most industrial systems.

Science does not know what energy is, but does know the accounting techniques for keeping track of it. Physics has constantly proven that energy cannot be created or called down from heaven or directly released by a magical pass of the hand, a *mantra*, a posture, a chant or an incantation. Any change that occurs in our world must be equated to an expenditure of a proportionate amount of energy from some other source. The process of physical change is measurable only by consideration of its status "before" and "after" and the amount of change equals the energy flow. Change is not free! The early founders of religion knew this law very well.

There are four major types of energy. The first type, called "entropic" energy, is the energy of the universe found in various manifestations such as fuel, wind, and solar radiation. This type of energy is gradually becoming less and less available as stars burn out and matter mixes together into one big homogeneous blob. For example, the center of the earth is cooling, mountains are wearing down, oil is being consumed, metal ores are becoming depleted and dispersed, arable land is decreasing, and soil is washing into the oceans.

The second type of energy called *prāna* which means "to bring forth breathing" or "vital energy," is that of biological processes in which a birth or rebirth replaces the decay of death. This natural biological energy is cyclical in that it goes through phases of creation, maturity, decay, death, and finally rebirth. *Prāna*, like entropic energy, can be found in several forms within the body such as within the basic energy of stimulated muscles, brain functions, and food digestion. *Prāna* in its highest form is stored as sexual energy and becomes the fuel for procreation as well as fuel for the even higher forms of individual energies, such as *shakti* and *kundalinī*.

The third type of energy called *shakti*[5] is limited to certain evolved humans who are able to leave behind more than their ashes or decaying bodies at death. Examples of what can remain are philosophical or religious developments, inventions, long-range constructions, new social concepts and changes, as well as personal changes which effect future lives including your own. This energy is associated with creations that survive the creator's death resulting in a reversal of the loss of energy or a gain in entropic energy. This type of energy brings more energy or intelligence into a world than had been there before.

The fourth type of energy called *kundalinī* is the evolutionary energy or the energy that allows a person to become something more than a programmed physical and mental body. This is the energy of transformation or liberation in which an individual is able to step into other worlds or dimensions. This is the energy that allows one to go beyond time or space and is the energy behind the mystical or religious experience.

The forces or powers referred to in *The Emerald Tablet* and the *Parātrimshikā* can be described as *shakti* and *kundalinī*. It must be recognized that these two energies or powers must be transformed from another source of energy or from the flow of energy in some other form. The modern investigations of energy have proven that energy can only be changed from one form to another and hence *shakti* has to be "paid for" with another source of energy. To the ancients, the source of energy for these creative and transcendent powers was from *prāna* that was stored as sexual energy or within organs located within the lower abdominal region.

The sexual energy of procreation as *prāna* was a very mystical power subject to a power beyond the individual. It should be noted that you cannot convert your normal physical or mental biological energy directly into *shakti* since a higher or compatible form of *prāna* energy is required. This can be compared to attempting to run your car on a cup of sugar or attempting to run a race on a glass of gasoline rather than a sugar drink. To the ancients the sexual energy had to be increased with sexual abstinence, proper physical practices, and proper mental practices (as will be described) with the basic *prāna* energy coming in from the proper diet and proper breathing. The practices, in other words, allowed the conversion of base biological energy or *prāna* obtained from food into *shakti* or a higher

---

[5] Defined as primal sexual energy in Chapter 7.

form of *prāna* energy. The *shakti* can then be converted into the even higher form of energy, *kundalinī*.

One of the body's processes of conversion of *prāna* to *shakti* is through "churning" of the lower abdomen that will be discussed in more detail in the next chapter and in *Part D* of this book. As a quick example of this conversion, you experience "gut wrenching" feelings before some challenge or demand. This "wrenching" can range from a mild tightening of the lower body in response to a nagging worry up to extreme wrenching during a hard crying or laughing session or in meeting the actual challenge. This wrenching is part of the natural body's energy conversion of *prāna* or sexual energy into *shakti*. You are conditioned, however, to suppress this "obscene," primitive and childish behavior and instead to tighten up the belly and take deep breaths. If you are facing an upcoming challenge such as facing your boss, you do not believe that you should get "uptight," worry, stew, or "get your guts in an uproar" and you then add your worry about the symptoms of worry to your total unrest. One solution to this problem is to engage in some activity that adds to the inner churning such as crying, moaning, rocking, dancing, deep exhalation, singing, walking or exercising. In contrast to your conditioning, this inner churning of the abdomen is beneficial, natural, and required to increase the *shakti* and your ability to tackle difficult challenges or problems.

The problem of describing and working with change can be stated as the problem of connecting two different realities together such as the "before" with the "after." The space between the "before" world and the "after" world is largely ignored in modern society, yet if one hopes to control change, then this *in-between* stage becomes very important. In terms of mental changes, it is not uncommon to find yourself suddenly in another mood or mindset without the awareness of the changing process of one to the other. Science faces a similar problem in the position of electrons around an atom when the atom either gives off energy or absorbs energy. The electrons do not gradually shift their positions, but do it instantaneously with an energy exchange. All biological changes are made up of this type of instant electron appearance-disappearance reactions with energy exchange.

In general, the "before" to the "after" change in which *shakti* is used takes place nearly instantly, as for instance, when you suddenly receive an answer to a complex question while you are in the shower. The changes involving *kundalinī* take place instantly outside of time as for instance

63

with the "near death experience" or spiritual visions or insights (*gnosis* or *jnāna*). However, with physical motion or growth so many atoms are generally required in a particular series that an observer sees a gradual shift in going from the "before" to the "after" as for instance in the flexing of a muscle in digging a hole.

This "before-world" to the "after-world" change can be described as a triad of:

1. the goal or change to be obtained (Sun element),
2. the energy or process to get there (Moon element), and
3. the final manifesting of the desired change (Heaven or manifested element).

For personal changes, one proceeds with a dedication which extends beyond any desires or specific results. In order to do this, one uses the creative process of *mantra* to be discussed in *Part B* using *shakti* generated by the techniques in *Part D*. The manifesting of change is through *mudrā* to be discussed in *Part C*.

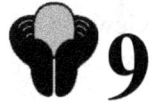

THE TRI-SEXUAL NATURE
OF THE BODY

"Of this it is certain, that as it is above, so it is below.
All things are from the One, by the One becoming Two."

The Emerald Tablet

The Gods (*Elohim*) said, "let *us* make man
in our image... male and female."

The Bible

"Those who do not have the existence of androgyny,
cannot break forth."

The Parātriṃshikā

There are many myths and religious stories about a single Creator of the universe who brings forth both male and female creatures. With this model, the Creator can be assumed to have been androgynous or to have had both masculine and feminine characteristics to pass on or to split off. The concept of androgynous Deities is therefore very common throughout the world in explaining the origin of the two sexes.

The developing Western world, however, required that the Creator be solely masculine. The opening statement of Genesis in the Bible (as quoted above) is typically ignored in favor of a following statement in Genesis stating that Elohim first created the man or Adam and then woman was created from Adam. This is interpreted to mean that Adam is a part of creation who furnishes the feminine characteristics rather than Elohim. With this questionable logic, Elohim can remain the strong patriarchal figure unadulterated with anything female. The patriarchal Western religions can also go further to separate Adam (and hence all men) from the female attributes by having those attributes (in the form of Eve) removed or cut out by Elohim. This operation after the creation of Adam then furnished the support for the religious lawyers to argue patriarchal or masculine

65

superiority that has deeply permeated the Western society ever since. This view also denies any aspect of androgyny or physical similarities of the two sexes since surgery separated the two.

Because of the Western religion-based negation of any aspect of androgyny and the complete separation of the male and female, several very important aspects about your sexual nature have been lost or suppressed over the centuries. The modern world believes that sexual function and nature are completely formulated and known by churches and by science. This is generally true about the reproductive system of humans. Great effort has been expended in studying sexual intercourse, and as a result sex has become a big business with the rise of many specialists in various aspects of reproductive sex ranging from problems of sexual impotency to promises of increased pleasure in intercourse. Science does know, however, that sexual characteristics do not quite fit the "either male or female" religious model. Science is well aware of the many variations in sexual response as well as variations in the physiology of sex organs including androgyny.

Both sexes are known to contain the opposite sex hormones (despite the religious concepts to the contrary) and their ratio can vary in the fetus producing androgynous characteristics as well as the individual sexual characteristics in infants. These androgynous characteristics are quickly surgically altered to produce normality and then further shifted, if required, with the administration of hormones. Any variation in the Biblical interpretation of gender is still taboo in the Western culture (as well in other patriarchal cultures).

There is, however, a change that can take place after puberty and this can be called the "third sex" because it is androgynous in that it has two sexual characteristics. As will be explained, this androgynous nature is but a continuation and further development of the initial or "primal" sexual energy of the prepubescent child. The re-experiencing of this primal sex is described in terms of having both the male and female sensations and reactions as will be described later. It is no doubt this experience of androgyny that is behind many unusual religious stories, practices, and images.

For example, the concept of androgyny is quite evident in some religious stories. The early Christians, for instance, described the religious experience with the male worshipper entering the bridal chamber (as a female) while mystics have used similar sexual metaphors in describing the encounter with the Divine. In his poem *Dark Night of the Soul*, Saint John of the Cross states that he went forth by a secret ladder when his house (body) was at rest (meditation) to where his lover (male) was awaiting him, and he ends being lost among the lilies without any cares. This is quite a vivid allegory to describe the deep sexual-like feelings aroused with the encounter of the Divine. This shift in sexual identity is common when individuals, both men and women, write about approaching the Divine.

The feminine religious garb in many Western religions and removal of beards are other reflections of the androgynous nature of the evolution of the body, which is noteworthy considering society's assertions as to the superiority of the masculine. This same confusion exists in the Eastern world which has many teachings of the female spiritual nature being supreme while again the male generally reigns supreme in the market-place.

A very unusual image of androgynous origin is found in the majority of Hindu temples.[6] This icon is a horizontal female pudendum or *yoni* with a protruding phallus coming out of the *yoni* called the *Shiva linga* (phallus). As will be described later, this protrusion of a *linga* from the *yoni* can actually be attained for varying periods of time by both men and women, with proper practices. In women, this protrusion is also accompanied with very strong masculine feelings and may be the basis for the concluding remark in the Gospel of Thomas that states, "Every woman who will make herself male will enter the kingdom of Heaven." Similarly, there are practices that produce very feminine androgynous characteristics in men that will be described shortly. In general, there are many men and women who find confusion with their gender identification when they experience awakening sensations of an androgynous nature.

One common thread through many cultures is the description of an inner flow of some form of power or energy that leads to transcendent or mystical experiences. In many cultures this flow is described in sexual terms or allegories which can be explained because of the intense lower sensations in the *yoni*. In particular, all of the major *Tantrik* writings consider that the source of all of the energies for the body and mind lies

---

[6] See Frontispiece.

within the lower part of the body in the "heart" or *yoni*, and specifically in the perineal or sexual region of the body.

Briefly, the primal sexual energy or *shakti* is the energy found in prepubescent children that assists in their ability to learn vicariously, to imagine or mentally create, and to play and communicate verbally with others. The primal sexual nature is quite obvious once you change your conditioned thinking about sex. You experienced it as a child with perineal pressure or massage, such as the very good feelings you found by sliding along a tree limb on your crotch, by putting pressure on the perineum, or by sleeping with your hands or a pillow in between your thighs. A young child loves perineal pressure and thinks rubbing is even better. What child does not love to ride your foot as a "horsie"? Likewise, is there a child who does not also love riding a tricycle that puts pressure against the perineal region as well as the massaging between the thighs and against the seat as the child pedals and moves?

Children love touching and being touched. We can quite easily visualize children squirming with pleasure as they are stroked or loved, or vibrating in anticipation of some cookies or candy. We remember them losing themselves completely in some game or in reacting with other children and how they seem to respond in unison in some of their seemingly weird and wild imaginative games. In play, they enjoy falling or being hit in the sexual region such as dropping to the ground during such games as "Ring Around the Rosie" (which of course gets even more exciting if they are aware of the symbolism of developing a rash and then dropping dead of the plague). They love their bodies and love to have close body contact with others. Recent studies demonstrate the remarkable increase in growth and learning if a young child is stroked and loved, and the lack of development or even death in infants when this is lacking. Remarkable improvements have been claimed with disturbed or retarded children riding bareback on horses, which amounts to direct stimulation of the perineum. It is not difficult to relate the normal child's rapid early growth to the primal sexual or perineal stimulation. It is no doubt because of this early sexual energy that many religious teachings point to the child as an example for learning the higher principles or as an example of the attainment of the higher realms of religion.

This primal energy or *shakti* is not found in animals and is generally suppressed by modern societies as the child matures. However, this energy can be refound and increased with special practices leading to a heightened response to others and the world. The supernormal experiences resulting from this increased *shakti* can range from the case of the small woman who lifts a car off of a pinned child, to the highly creative outputs of motivated individuals.

With the activation of *shakti* or the further development of the primal sex, there is a shift in your center of being. The average Westerner believes the center of being to be in the middle of the head because of the intense discipline and the conditioned usage of the brain with its judgement and analysis. This can be contrasted with the average Easterner or primitive who identifies the center of being as within the chest because of the conditioning in the East as to the importance of feelings and trust. As the Westerner increases the *shakti*, the perceived center of the Self lowers within the body. With the development of androgyny, the center of being drops to the lower gut or sexual region that is called the center, heart, fire, or a heating cauldron, etc. in the mystical schools.

Some of the characteristics of the flow of *shakti* are well known within the modern society. For instance, many individuals have reported the incredible rise of "imagination" during sexual intercourse while they were reaching for an orgasm. Along with this highly active imagination in which their partner might become the most beautiful person in the world is the complete loss of ego. Many people suffer what is called a "global amnesia" in which they lose much of their conditioned responses and memory of such things as their partner's name (which can be embarrassing of course!) One obvious conclusion about the so-called "near death" experience is the lack of concern or fear that you are dead. This state of mind, although not mentioned in most reports, would seem to be the most shocking since you would think that finding yourself dead would really be upsetting. The sense of ecstasy, of being in a new world and body, of possessing higher powers of mind and body, of having no fears or concerns, are but some of the effects of the flow of *shakti*.

The mystical schools used allegories in describing the rising of the creative energy (*shakti*) within the body. Alchemy depicted it as upward progressing reactions within the athanor and thinly veiled its descriptions with the substitution of lead for the basic energy of the body (*prāna*) and gold for the results of the upward flowing evolutionary forces. Christianity described this process in terms of the rising of the inner "spirit" or quickening force. Certainly, the evolution of an individual is a far greater miracle than converting lead into gold or converting water into wine or even healing the body of illnesses.

The use of children in the old allegories also suggests the third sex or androgyny and the unique sexual nature of *shakti*. Alchemical artwork, for instance, many times depicts a young prepubescent boy and girl in a mock sexual embrace, while the New Testament of the Bible has several references to the advantages of being like a child. References to childhood can stimulate the wonderful feelings of the body without the distraction of the sexual drive and allow the assimilation of the concept of a higher force of unification.

One of the earliest expositions on the sexual forces was through the *Tantrik* writings in India which were later carried throughout the known world including Egypt, which was described as one of the spiritual centers at the time of Jesus. Buddhism is known to have carried the *Tantrik* concepts of the sexual source throughout the East where they became merged with local models and ideas. The Chinese *Taoist* teachings are clear in speaking of the lower fires in the body and the stimulation of the sex to increase the inner flow of *shakti* called *chi* which was later called *ki* by the Japanese.

Before starting with the physical sources of the higher sexual forces, it is necessary to speak first of pleasure particularly since you are conditioned to be afraid of deep inner pleasure other than that of sexual orgasm (for procreation.) The materialistic and puritanical West assumes that seeking pleasure interferes with duty and calls this hedonism, which is a derogatory term in our modern world. The Puritanical school believed that suffering was good for character, while the modern Liberals in opposing puritanical thinking like to believe that while suffering is bad, hedonism or excessive joy and ecstasy are also bad or at least highly suspect. Both schools manage to make everyone who seeks ecstasy a possible social deviant. The system of *Tantra*, however, teaches that one of the main reasons that you exist is for *kāma*, which means pleasure as well as the desire and yearning for more and more pleasure.

The practices that stimulate the primal sexual energies lead into the capability of experiencing joy as the lower abdomen is freed from constraint and tension. It should be noted that the same primal energy also liberates the brain from some of the conditioning it has undergone and allows you to think more clearly. *Kāma* is not the normal pleasure of being good, or of attaining a specific goal, nor is it the pleasure of a sexual orgasm (despite the popularity of a book from India called the *Kāma Sutra* that is about sexual play). *Kāma* is close to Freud's concept of "libido" being a basic driving force except that it is not interpreted to be limited to the sexual drive.

Kāma is the reaching for more and more pleasure, and therefore *kāma* can never be satisfied. For instance, reaching for a sexual orgasm is *kāma*, but at orgasm there is cessation of *kāma*. One of the basic objects that you seek is some form of pleasure that goes beyond what you have already experienced. You have a desire to find a special absorbing closeness with others that has not yet been experienced or you feel that there is never enough within any relationship. In sexual interactions you yearn for something that is more continual, more a merging together and uniting in some intense pleasure. In the marketplace, it is reaching for more and more abilities, interactions, or challenges and it is always beyond you.

Kāma is the process of attempting to fulfill that which is yearned for. It is a process and not that which is being sought. An example is given with the difference between romantic love and mature love. Romantic love is reaching for more and more closeness and union that requires effort and the experiencing of intense *kāma*. Mature love is fulfilled love without change or *kāma* and is typified by the lack of reaching for more love or new experiences or by the lack of union. The majority of people are satisfied with mature love, but who doesn't sometimes wish for romantic love?

Our modern culture teaches us to be satisfied, controlled, conforming, and secure with what we have. *Tantrik* students face a very strong opposition as they attempt to feel more and more pleasure or to obtain *kāma*. They were taught by society to believe that this is sinful (for some unknown reason,) and that it will turn into something bad, or that they will lose control of themselves and do something terrible. The Westerner is deeply ingrained with guilt and avoidance of anything new. You have experienced this many times as you start to lose yourself in some situation that becomes more and more pleasurable until you become frightened of some vague possible consequences. These uneasy feelings are generally of the form that you will have to pay for this with some deep suffering that will catch up with you later.

There are centers within the body for controlling *kāma* and hence the production of the complex biochemicals that control or stimulate the functioning of the body, but society teaches and enforces postures, tensions, thoughts, and breathing which suppress these centers. The intensity of *kāma* is determined by the control centers that are further modified by the activity within the *yoni*.

The word *yoni* has a number of meanings with the most common being the sexual organ of a female. It has also the meanings of being a source or center of life and as such is also called the *hridaya*, which is generally translated as "heart" (which gives problems to most translators). The word *yoni* comes from a root which means "to unite" (*yu*), so it is the organ of union or the coupling between the "I" and the "You" or the "That." This *yoni* is also considered to be the central connection of the *nādis* of the body that serves to couple the *tattvas* both within and outside the body. This will be discussed in detail in Chapter Eleven dealing with the *Tattvas* and *Chakras*.

The word *yoni* in modern *Sanskrit* usage has both a masculine and feminine gender associated with it, but in the early *Rig Veda* writings before 500 BC, it had only the masculine connotation. The writings of *Yoga* describe and locate the *yoni* (in men) quite clearly as: "it is like a mouth or opening that resides behind the base of the penis and in front of the anus. It is found with a depth equal to the distance across four fingers, and it is hidden with a covering of a cloth like material." (Some writings refer to the *yoni* as "the hidden" or *guhya*.) Despite this clear description, the *yoni* is largely ignored since the modern world "knows" that men do not have such an opening, hidden or not. Some scholars assume, however, that when the *yoni* is referred to, it means related to *yoginīs* or female *yogis*. This referral is perhaps more accurate, since as will be discussed, *yogis* can develop the female characteristics and in some literature such as the *Parātrimshikā*, male *yogis* who have mastered the practices are clearly referred to as *yoginīs*.

The *yoni* occupies a fairly large space that includes the volume bounded by the perineal skin, behind the front pubic arch, the anus, and the lower abdominal wall. In women it is found in the same region and includes the vagina and the surrounding muscles. The perineal region of Western men is normally quite hard, tough, and impenetrable and many men after hearing about the *yoni*, will quickly deny its existence since they cannot find any opening or even any soft tissue. However, after prolonged stretching and exercising, it becomes soft and then a finger can easily probe into it. Once the *yoni* is softened, the above ancient description in the *Yoga* writings can be understood. A finger will penetrate until it reaches the deep layer of the superficial fascia or the support for the forward abdominal area which, in the forward area of the perineum, has a depth of about the distance of the width of four fingers. As the *yoni* becomes fully activated it can feel like a lower mouth as described in *Yoga* writings.

The *yoni* essentially disappears when it is not activated or sensitized in that the softness and openness disappear and the perineum return to normal. It is this behavior of the *yoni* that keeps it out of the physiology books, since it certainly is not evident on a corpse or the average non-stimulated patient undergoing an examination by a medical doctor.

The development of the *yoni* is first begun in general with the stretching of the perineal skin and supporting tissue. This stretching is fundamental to most of the Eastern disciplines. Almost without exception the martial arts, *Hathayoga,* and other popular *Yoga* are taught with the students in sitting postures with the legs crossed and thighs extended for lengthy periods. It is certain that most teachers could not explain the persistence of this practice although the explanation is very simple in terms of the development of the *yoni*. The standard meditating posture of *Yoga* is a very easy method of stretching the tissue and ligaments of the perineum such that the *yoni* can expand and open in men as well as women. The descriptions of the proper material to sit upon in the early *yogic* writings (such as a tiger skin on dried manure) serve to also bring pressure to the *yoni* for further stimulation. Without this type of stretching as well as the other practices associated with the *yoni*, the *yoni* cannot be penetrated and remains fully hidden.

The first indication of the existence of the *yoni* in men can be found by inserting a finger into the middle of the scrotum to pick up loose flesh and then moving the finger towards the anus sliding it under the perineal skin until an opening of the *yoni* can be felt or entered. Later the perineal region changes such that the finger can be directly inserted into the *yoni* through the perineum without much opposition. Women notice the shift in sensitivity and tenderness with pressure around the labia. It should be noted that the *yoni* in men does not have a hole such as the vagina, but rather softens to such an extent that a finger can be inserted into it.

The development of the *yoni* is described within *Part D* of this book. The listed practices develop the lower abdominal muscles long unused since early childhood and introduce methods for the internal stimulation of the *yoni* with churning of the lower muscles and use of the breathing muscles and breath. The churning is similar to that found in belly and exotic dancing in which the lower abdominal muscles are used independently to cause the agitated motion of the lower abdomen. This becomes stimulating both to the observer as well as the dancer. In contrast to these exercises, our culture teaches everybody to tighten their bellies and to tuck their fannies under, to take deep breaths, to pull the tummies in and never to allow sexual-like motions of the body. You are also conditioned to keep your anus and sexual muscles tight to prevent "leakages." All of these prohibit the *yoni* from responding and evolving.

As the *yoni* is further stimulated, a swelling occurs within the *yoni* that is called the *kanda* which means "bulb or chord." Initially the swelling is very subtle in that it expands without much pressure, that is, as the *kanda* starts to swell it can readily be suppressed with a very light countering pressure. To the fingers, the *kanda* initially feels as if it is filled with a very soft gel or foam with little form. As it develops, it becomes firmer and takes on a definite tube or bulb shape. This bulb ultimately extends from the base of the penis in men and from the bottom edge of the pubic arch in women (same position in both sexes) toward the anus or vagina and then inward and upwards.

The *kanda* lies behind the front of the pubic bone structure and in front of the vagina (or that location if you had a vagina.) With swelling, a further increase in sensitivity of the perineum occurs when the perineum is very lightly stroked. The swelling is obvious in men and can be physically observed where it can become larger than a one-inch diameter bulb or tube extending from the base of the penis even though the penis and base are not enlarged. The *kanda* is initially more hidden in women by the labia that normally swells as well, but the protruding of the total pudendum becomes quite pronounced with swelling equal to that in men with proper excitation or stimulation of the *kanda*.

In women, as the *kanda* becomes swollen and firm, the vagina is pressed shut and penetration into it with a penis can become difficult. The swelling can press outward through the opening of the vagina which is the basis for several distorted dictionary definitions. For example, *kanda* is defined as "(is like) uteri prolapses or the protrusion of the uterus from the vagina." Another description calls it *yonyarsha* which means "(like a) hemorrhoid of the *yoni*." This development can terrify many if they have not been told to expect it and may deter them from continuing the practices that produce it. You can easily verify that the uterus has not fallen with the insertion of a finger into the vagina. You will find instead very healthy and strong support for the uterus from the developed pelvic floor muscles and well developed sexual and urethra muscles, if the outlined practices have been followed. The strengthening of these muscles and increased blood flow is also known to prevent or alleviate vaginal disorders.

As the *yoni* becomes more and more active your center of awareness drops from the middle of your head to the area of the *yoni* which is why it is also called the heart. As this center of being is transferred, the reliance upon thinking diminishes as "feelings" are found to be more reliable and exciting. The old writings speak of the generation of *soma* or an "unseen fertile fluid" from the lower heart or *yoni*, and this may be explained in today's science as the production of powerful neuropeptides, hormones, or other bio-chemicals which have an immediate as well as a long-range effect on the body.

Many individuals who had experienced drug "rushes" before the *Tantrik* practices, report that the rise of this inner fluid feels very similar but far better than the drug rush. It is also referred to as the "golden womb" in old writings because of the intense feelings and awareness that the *yoni* becomes the source for a new or "quickened" life. The *yoni* is also considered to be the central connection point for all of the *nādis* that link the *tattvas*. (See next chapter.) The *nādis* are likened to the nerves of the body but are better considered as an interconnecting system of conduits like the lymph system.

In both sexes, the excitation of the developed and opened *yoni* and *kanda* is far more stimulating and pleasing than that of the clitoris or penis (although they remain as sensitive as before). One difference with this third type or primal sex is that it requires increasing muscular effort and concentration to maintain or to increase the pleasure. It is much different from sex where the sexual drive takes over, and the body responds "automatically" as contrasted with the strong conscious and physical effort required with the primal response. Only after prolonged practicing can you notice the swelling of the *kanda* with relatively normal demands on the body or mind without conscious effort or control.

As the sensitivity increases and controlling muscles are developed, it becomes easier to activate the *yoni* with simple practices such as lower abdominal breathing (or use of the lower lung capacity to breathe.) As the perineum region becomes more sensitive, a deep exhalation forces the *levator ani* muscle to push air out of the lungs to move and to stimulate the *yoni*. Sitting in meditation for very long and repeated sessions can also stimulate the *yoni*, as for instance reported by a recent popular writer on *kundalinī*, Gopi Krishna. He wrote that his first awakening to *kundalinī* started after very long hours of meditation when suddenly he felt a sensation "…so extraordinary and so pleasing…at the place touching the seat…" Women report similar experiences during prolonged sexual foreplay where the *yoni* becomes physically stimulated.

When the *kanda* is active there are changes in the mind and body that can be alarming if not understood. The activity of the *kanda* has the net result of opening you to an expanded and created world that includes what would normally be considered as religious. You accept the presence of a guiding hand in your life or in the magic of the game of life. You are aware of the power in your own dedication, Will, *shakti*, and the power of the body and mind. The body feels more supple and sensual with the rising of wonderful feelings in the *yoni*. The body feels tender and gentle which adds to your expanded world. In the modern Western culture such changes are associated with the feminine nature and it becomes of concern to the average male who has been conditioned to be "macho." There are, however, other changes that can be interpreted as masculine such as the rise in self-confidence, sense of power and control, as well as keener insight. These traits can be of concern to a woman who has been conditioned to be timid, shy, and removed from the responsibilities of the marketplace. These changes can be misinterpreted into an even more limited view of your sexual gender rather than into an acceptance of having both sexual traits or of becoming androgynous.

When the *kanda* becomes active another change can occur which is called the rise of the *kundalinī*. This change is related to an inner organ called the *Shiva linga* or the phallus of the God *Shiva*. This *linga* is described as projecting downward toward the perineum with its base against the floor of the abdominal wall or the *svadhistana chakra* region. The ancient description states that around the *Shiva linga* is coiled a serpent called the *kundalinī*. When properly stimulated, the serpent uncoils and darts toward the base of the spine and hammers against the "sacred" sacrum bone until it is able to penetrate the bone and then find its way up the center of the spine to the interior of the head. This description is a model which describes the experiences of many people who find it easy to envision a serpent banging against the sacrum when the advanced disciplines are being learned. As mentioned before, the Hindus use an icon called the *Shiva linga* in their temples, which was no doubt correlated originally with the physical experiences of the further activation of the *kanda*.

The precursor to the rising of the serpent is felt within men and women as certain of the practices or *mahāsādhanas* are being done. This feeling is associated with the development of something growing within the *yoni* that is more than the swelling *kanda*. If inner body pressure is applied to the growth, a protrusion of something relatively hard and with a phallus-like shape is felt being forced out through the surface tissues. This feeling is generally pleasant and might be compared with defecation. Others report the feeling of a rupture although it also feels good. This protrusion extends beyond the perineum and can best be described as appearing as the Hindu icon with a phallus coming forth from a female pudendum.

It is this appearance of the *Shiva linga* that opens into another world of sexual-like responses and body-mind changes. This protrusion of the *Shiva linga* is difficult to maintain and can instantly disappear if the concentration of the practices is disturbed. Some of the old writings describe this *linga* as being very "shy" which is an excellent description. The appearance of the *Shiva linga* with the sense of "rupturing" yourself can be of great concern when it first occurs, but as everything can quickly revert back to normal, the anxieties can be controlled, particularly if you find that your normal sex is unchanged. In fact, your pelvic floor and inner muscles are far healthier as discussed in Chapter Twenty-three.

The *Shiva linga* is so called, because it is related to the creative power of the Sun or of the "masculine" force. The *linga* normally extends during advanced practices as mentioned or also during intense pleasure with, for instance, the physical union of two *yonis* or in some outer demand upon the mind or body which requires special supernormal powers. For instance, some people report the intense and strong sexual-like fatigue in the groin following some extreme trauma when they have exerted supernormal powers.

One of the practices used in finding the *kanda* uses the stimulation of the nipples with other exercises. The majority of people are instantly repelled with the idea of nipple stimulation, which is of course, simply the result of social conditioning. In men and women connections are to be found between the nipples of the breast and the *yoni* or *kanda*. The two nipples are described as the Sun and the Moon in ancient literature and are connected with the more popular concept of the heating and cooling natures of the two sides of the body or of the *ida* and *pingala nādis*. As the *yoni* and *kanda* develop, the sensitivity of the nipples likewise increases. As you massage the nipples, a corresponding pleasurable feeling is or can be obtained in the *yoni*.

Some women have experienced this connection following childbirth when they felt pleasurable contractions in the uterus and vagina during nursing. However, many of these women were horrified and suppressed the wonderful feelings when they interpreted the feelings as sexual, and evidencing some perverse psychological feelings toward their child. Most men are conditioned from an early age to ignore and suppress feelings in their nipples. Also, since most men are concerned for their self-image as males, they similarly repress any sensitivity or connections to the *yoni*. That this connection or functioning of the nipples is not known is evidenced by the simple observation that in the modern world it is acceptable for men to show their nipples, whereas women may not. In a small sample of men and women, it appeared that about half of the men and women could report that nipple stimulation felt good, although after mastering the advanced practices, everyone found the wonderful feelings and connections to the *yoni*.

The primal sex or the hidden sex cannot co-exist with the reproductive sexual responses; however, they may be switched back and forth even after mastery of the *Shiva linga*. As one response is achieved the other rapidly falls away. For instance, once the *yoni* is stimulated, both the clitoral and penile erections cease; however, light stimulation can further increase the stimulation of the *yoni* without stimulating the normal sexual responses. Also, the swelling *kanda* will tend to suppress penetration of a penis into the vagina. If, however, the reproductive sex is stimulated first, then the hidden sexual response does not appear. Both sexes experience the activation of the *yoni* as a change in gender response. The erection of the *Shiva lingam* is certainly perceived as masculine to females and the opening sensation and swelling of the *kanda* is perceived as very feminine to males. In fact, both sexes can equate the *kanda* excitation as being "super feminine."

With the energized *kanda,* a state of mind can be found in terms of your relationship with others or with the Divine that can only be described as oneness or union. This might be explained in common terms as "operating on the gut level," where you respond according to your feelings rather than to your thought processes. In this state of mind, you perceive the world as one large interaction with everything seeming to fit together in perfect harmony. You seem to have a deep understanding and union with others even though you may be acting in opposition to them in life situations. It is this state that allows you to play games with others or to respond promptly with the necessary physical or mental response to a crisis or demand.

With the increased production of *shakti,* the ancient references to the "Two Truths" become meaningful.[7] Dyads that were the basis for reality were called the "Two Truths" and included such pairs as:

- masculine and feminine,
- heating and cooling,
- creating and manifesting,
- evolution and involution,
- pleasure and duty,
- freedom and bondage.

Many of the ancient teachings are concerned with balancing these opposing forces. For instance, the English word "righteous" as used in the New Testament of the Bible means to be "balanced" or equal. As has been discussed in Chapter Four, social behavior is based upon the balance of "shoulds" and "should nots."

Both of the opposing forces are concentrated, formed or released from the sexual region as will be discussed in detail in Chapter Eleven. The masculine force is experienced as a deep yearning for more and new experiences originating in the groin, while the feminine is experienced as the desire to merge with, to become a part of someone or something, and first experienced in the groin and then the chest as it becomes manifested. Obviously, if a union is to be found, there must be the dedication for it as well as the manifesting or experiencing of it. In sexual terms, there must first be a strong attraction followed by the actual contact and union. In modern society both of these forces are suppressed; however, the ancient

---

[7] See Chapter 3.

teachings argue that both forces must be energized and coupled or balanced. This is required in order to reach the object of dedication and make it manifest or real.

You have had the experience of being strongly attracted to someone and then thoroughly enjoying being with them in a close or intimate sharing of thoughts, ideas, or experiences with very strong sexual-like feelings. Touching can further increase this and an intense union can be obtained with a specific partner without sexual orgasm. These experiences leave you feeling very much alive and aware afterward, rather than enervated and disinterested as following sexual orgasm. People who learn to activate their *kandas* report an almost constant sexual-like stimulation while observing attractive people of both sexes. They also tell of the intense joy associated with everyday personal interactions. In other words, to be fully alive you should have as much sexual stimulation and union as possible, but little or no sexual orgasms.

Some Near Eastern "wives' tales" spoke of a different type of sexual activity that the Sheiks learned to keep their harems of women happy. Similar tales abound with the *Tantriks* claiming that they had discovered the secrets of sexual orgasm and pleasure. There is in fact a strong basis for these tales; however, the activities do not employ a sexual orgasm nor the normal sexual excitation nor penetration. One descriptive term which the *Tantriks* used to describe this union or *maithuna*[8] was *kunda-golaka* which can be translated as "ball and socket." The *yonis* are brought into contact with specific postures.

One pose that has become a basis for many false claims involves two people sitting together with one in the other's lap. The assumption commonly made is that a woman is sitting on top of a man with prolonged penile penetration. Looking to experience this *Tantrik* union, many misguided seekers pay for fraudulent courses which supposedly teach how to maintain this assumed erect penile penetration for long periods of time. Certainly, the actual *Tantrik* sitting pose can be held for hours with intense ecstasy, but there is no penetration by the penis and neither the clitoris nor the penis is excited. Instead, the two *Shiva lingas* are stimulated which are then directed to protrude against the yielding flesh of the partner and join similar to two ball and socket joints. Since the flesh is soft, the *Shiva lingas* are partially formed by the partner and displaced such that both are shaped,

---

[8] See Chapter 20.

move, and project into the right places. Needless to say, the non-*Tantriks* will not attain this posture or its results from any weekend course.

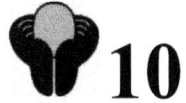

10
SOMA

"The junction of the two *Tantrik* powers
brings forth all of the powers in the form of
a flowing unseen creative fluid (*soma*)."

The Parātrimshikā

"Imbibe *soma* for mighty power and vigor."

The Rig Veda

The oldest religious writing in the world is about *soma* and is contained in ten books called the *Rig Veda*. The title means "Hymns of Knowledge" and had its origin in about 1000 BC. The books were written by "Aryans" living in the Indus Valley of India about whom very little is known. The books in general are about Gods and how *soma* gives them powers. There are considerable descriptions of both the source of *soma* and its preparation although both are very imprecise. The most accepted explanation of *soma* offered by today's writers is that it was prepared from some psychedelic plant using prescribed ritualistic tools in a ceremonial ritual. This explanation has absolutely no support, however, since no drawings or detailed descriptions of the plant can be found and no known plant has the very broad medicinal properties ascribed to *soma*. Another problem is that the writings are very contradictory when they are applied to the characteristics and processing of a plant. There is, however, considerable support for the *yoni* being the source of *soma* as described in the *Parātrimshikā*.

The verses of the *Rig Veda* are quite compatible with the *Parātrimshikā* when it is understood that the descriptions many times are based on feelings associated with the churning activity around the *yoni*. Another strong support for this interpretation is that among the few artifacts found in the ancient Aryan communities were a large number of icons of the *yoni* and *Shiva linga*. These icons, as has been mentioned, are still used in Hindu temples, although the original meanings of these icons appear to have been lost over the centuries. When the references and descriptions of the *Rig Veda* are accepted as allegorical and related to individual experiences instead of to Gods and forces outside of the Self, deeper meanings

83

can be obtained. For instance, each God described in the books can be seen to be symbolic of inner feelings and forces.

The overall message of the books can therefore be considered as a testimonial on the effort required to generate *soma* and *soma's* power in overcoming many of the inner weaknesses. The last book of the *Rig Veda* states that all of the Gods came from the "One," again in keeping with the other writings. The last book also denies that *soma* comes from the crushing and pressing of a plant, but rather is an inner "God." One very important consideration is that the *Rig Veda* is like the Sermon on the Mount of the Bible, in that it can only have meaning to the select few who have opened to and experienced the inner powers. To the remainder it remains an inspiration or as a promise of something greater.

The word *soma* is used over one thousand times in the *Rig Veda* in reference to the creative and powerful fluid. Some of the prominent traits ascribed to its use are: knowledge, bravery, strength, supernormal powers (*siddhis*), union with the (inner) gods, and compassion. A few selected verses from the *Rig Veda* about *soma* are:

> "...it makes you victorious and invincible and is intoxicating..."

> "...when you imbibe the *soma*, you become immortal..."

> "...with its light you can discover the Divine..."

> "*Soma* is a protection that must be allowed free flow through the body in order to break the bonds of illness and to couple the body tightly together."

These descriptions are also reminiscent of the drink of Ambrosia described in a later time by writers of the Greek and Roman gods.

The origin of *soma* is described in the *Rig Veda* as follows:

> "The source of *soma* is contained within the inner vault of Heaven and covers itself with a stretched cloth soft as a cloud."

> "It is produced from a swollen bulb like a swollen udder."[9]

---

[9] See Chapter 9 on the *kunda*.

"When milked with pressing and churning, the bulb is freed and the sweetness flows and mixes with the flowing waters (fluids of the body) and flows throughout the world (body)."

The source of *soma* is sometimes related to a milk cow such as "flowing forth from the cow in Heaven" and might have been the source of the Hindu worship of the cow. Other terms used in its preparation include pounding, drawing, squeezing, lifting, pouring, and filtering, all which describe the feelings produced by advanced *yogic* practices as outlined in Chapter Twenty-three.

The *Parātriṃshikā* gives the keys to unlocking the mystery of where *soma* is produced and its effects. However, it does not give the method of the production of *soma*. When the keys offered by the definitions of the *Parātriṃshikā* are applied to other Indian documents the story of *soma* becomes complete. A common statement in old writings in many cultures is concerned with the conversion of sexual fluids into a more refined powerful fluid. *Sanskrit* describes this process with the term *ūrdhva retas*, or the upward flow of a fluid. This fluid is mistakenly assumed to be a refined or altered form of semen or sexual fluid transformed into the form of *soma*, and this misconception prevail in most modern Indian schools (and also in other cultures) who decry the loss of semen in sexual orgasm without procreation.

One of the highly recommended esoteric practices of India provides the clue to the pounding, pressing, pulling, and filtering described in the *Rig Veda* for preparing *soma*. This practice is called *mantham* or churning and it is easy to find references to it although the details are not readily available. This practice will be discussed in Chapters Twenty-two and Twenty-three. In general, churning consists of using the lower abdominal muscles in such a way that the *yoni* and *kanda* are stimulated. (It is interesting to mention here that some men report a similar deep inner pounding sensation and churning preceding the nocturnal emission.) As the *kanda* becomes swollen it feels like a "swollen bulb or udder" and there is the great desire to "milk" it or to pull up the contents. Another Indian model is that the *yoni* becomes as a lower mouth. This model can be coupled with other practices that suggest sucking up from the *yoni* to yield the model of a thirsty mouth sucking up *soma*.

The production of *soma* and the amount of *soma* produced is dependent upon the stimulation or need. *Soma* is something like a universal hormone that stimulates the body and mind such that they can better approach any demand. For instance, in the case of the woman lifting a car off of a child, the *soma* may function as a muscle stimulant and pain suppressant. In the case where increased mental function is required, *soma* may take a form that stimulates the brain and sensory organs. *Soma* is the fuel for the special mentally controlled powers called *siddhis* that function to manifest complete fulfillment of that which is required to reach the dedicated goal. (It should be stressed that *soma* cannot be produced to satisfy personal desires.)

One of the first physical characteristics to be changed with *soma* is the reaction time of the body. The first martial artists are generally believed to have been *yogis* who had mastered *Tantra*. When the *soma* flows one may experience the state of suspended time that has been reported by athletes and others during trauma where there are severe demands upon the mind and body. The response time of the nerves and muscles is at least doubled.[10] With suspended time, increased awareness, and enhanced mental and physical capabilities, it is easy to be victorious against an opponent. The secret of the martial arts is the production of *soma* or the state of mind and body that produces it.

The selection of what powers are to be manifested or enhanced by *soma* certainly does not exist at the conscious level and must come forth from a more subtle or at the Soul level. Physiologists and psychologists already know how the subconscious mind can vary hormones and other biochemicals produced by the body. Intense trauma is known to produce wide variations in the biochemical production of the body as the body is prepared to respond well beyond its normal capabilities. The sensation of pleasure is many times preceded by the sensation of an upward flowing fluid found to be dependent upon the generation of a neurotransmitter called dopamine. *Soma* can therefore be assumed to be generated in order to stimulate the body and mind like processes controlled by some of the known natural biochemicals. Unlike other body biochemicals, however, *soma* is capable of freeing the Self from the identification with the bondage of social conditioning as well as providing increased strength and mental abilities.

As *soma* flows, the conditioned brain quiets and the socially imposed inhibitions disappear. This is sufficient to equate *soma* with normal intox-

---

[10] See Appendix A, *Response Time for Tantriks.*

ication, but there is also extreme euphoria, ecstasy, and union with others. The temporary losses of ego, fear, and memory have already been discussed. *Tantriks* can play and relate together as perhaps only creative and free children can do. Critics of *Tantra* and the *Rig Veda* could very well use their impression of intoxicated *Tantriks* to describe them as evil people intoxicated upon some unholy brew. It is interesting that the same criticism was leveled against some of the early Christians during their "love feasts" and that Jesus was also accused as being a winebibber. However, the Bible contains descriptions of substances that are no doubt the equivalent of *soma*. For example, within the book of John the "living water" is certainly similar to the *Rig Veda* speaking of *soma*. The Book of John states that the living water springs up into everlasting life and flows forth out of the belly of a believer. This can be compared to a number of statements in the *Rig Veda* about *soma* giving immortality to those who imbibe.

The excitement of the *kanda* and *Shiva linga* can be considered as contagious. There is an increased sensitivity within your own *yoni* that is found in the presence of others with excited *yonis*. There is enhanced group empathy when the *kandas* are active and *soma* is being produced. The groups can quickly respond to higher emotions and experiences during common worship, singing, dancing, or playing. The "songs" in the *Rig Veda* may well have been impromptu creations during such gatherings. It is noted that very expressive insights can be obtained during the sharing of *soma* and that a leader can find the knowledge necessary to lead a group further toward their common goal or dedication. Some fundamentalist groups around the world approach this same enhanced group dynamics as they surrender themselves to a higher power and allow a common "game" to take place. As the *vimarsha* increases, so does the flow of *shakti* or *soma* and the state of intoxication or *madya* is approached.

PART B

THE SUN OR THE CREATIVE REALM

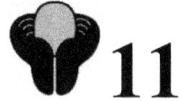

11

THE PHYSICAL
TO SUBTLE CONNECTIONS

"For as he thinketh in his heart, so is he."

The Bible

"Tell me of this hidden aspect of myself
which shines forth largely unhidden."

The Parātriṃshikā

This chapter is primarily concerned with the connection between the subtle and the physical or how thoughts can affect the physical feelings or vice versa. For instance, you are aware of how your feelings can affect your health, such as when you perceive a frown from your boss that in turn sets up tensions, loss of sleep, and then a cold. You also sense a relationship with how your day goes depending upon the mood you wake up with. If you wake up with the feelings of gloom and doom, everything in your world turns gloomy.

A model that is currently being used by science to explain this coupling of the unmanifest forces to the manifest is that certain organs or sites within the body secrete or release complex chemicals as a result of being stimulated with either the brain or senses. These biochemicals in turn travel to other organs or sites which then changes the overall functioning of the body and brain. A simple example of this is the release of adrenaline from the adrenal glands in the abdominal region with fear. It is interesting that the early *Tantrik* researchers derived another model that is very similar at least functionally to the modern scientific thinking. This earlier model does have the advantage that is serves as a tool in learning to control the inner processes and correlates with personal feelings and experiences.

Table 1 in *Part E* contains all of the pieces used in the *Tantrik* model. This model is based upon active centers, called *tattvas*, that can be considered to work similarly to the inner controlling organs in the modern concept described above. You may well argue the actual reality of most of the *tattvas* as well as their placement, and it should be noted that different *Tantrik* schools do not agree on their locations and functions either.

The *Tantrik* model of the Self consists of five chief levels that can be listed in order from the subtle to the gross as follows:

Levels		*Tantrik* Model of the Self	
I		**Inner Creators**	Masculine and Feminine Forces (Sun and Moon)
	Subtle		
II		**Pre-Spirit**	The initial separation from the eternal and unmanifest.
III		**Spirit**	The defining and contraction of Self and world.
IV		**Soul**	The subtle or preliminary mental manifesting of Self.
	Gross		
V		**Self**	Expansion into the outer world or the manifested being.

The Pre-Spirit stage is the interface between the totality of the Self as Nothingness and the awareness of Self and non-Self things. This stage has been discussed in terms of the experience of waking from a deep sleep into an unknown world.

The Pre-Spirit can be compared with the life force that exists behind all living matter. Only its growth can be physically described and that growth can be ascribed to an inner force or Will.

The Pre-Spirit, after starting to become "cohesive" and grasping a sense of consciousness as in shaking loose from a deep sleep, becomes labeled as Spirit which forms the basics of the Self and outer world. The Spirit sets the spirit, flavor, and color of the world to be created. This Spirit may also be compared to the DNA structure within your body. The DNA carries the basic blueprints or program for the organization of your body and your basic traits. Each person's DNA structure is unique although it carries hereditary traits as well. The formation of the DNA molecule limits as well as defines the body and mind which will be built by its own plan. The organization of the DNA molecule or Spirit can be assumed to have been selected, controlled, or held by the Pre-Spirit or basic life force.

The Soul furnishes the detailed description of the world and Self and how it is to be experienced. The Soul creates what can be called the dream as well as experiences the created dream.

There are some important questions that need to be addressed before continuing.

- How does the Soul communicate with the physical Self?

- How can a thought produce a feeling?

- How can a strong mood or feeling in someone else produce the same mood or feeling within you?

The answer to these questions lies in the nature of vibrations. There is a basic phenomenon in physics that objects tend to resonate or vibrate together. This effect is enhanced if the objects have nearly the same frequencies of vibration. This is extended to the "feelings" or vibrations in people such as you might say, "two people resonate together," meaning they are able to "feel" the same things.

Humans are the only species that are known to be cognizant of continuous vibration and able to produce physical vibrations of a resonating nature. Birds may fly in formation to minimize air resistance, but they do not flap their wings in unison. Horses run together but not in step and cannot be trained to do so. Whales make noises called singing, but they do not have a rhythm and do not make noises together in unison or harmony. Cows may be soothed with the noise of music but they do not respond to the rhythm. Cows simply do not swish their tails or nod their heads in time with the music. Animals cannot be taught to dance or respond to the rhythm of music. Animals can create sounds used in basic communication

93

such as warnings or mating calls, but only humans are capable of resonating together and developing further resonances.

Humans are sensitive to gross physical rhythms such as a drumbeat or the beat in music. Humans are also able to synchronize movements to a rhythm such as in marching in step or working in synchronism on an assembly line. It is recognized that a regular beat or rhythm can have direct effects upon your inner energies. It is not as well recognized, however, in our highly regulated society, that an irregular beat or rhythm can be even more powerful.

For instance, a witch doctor can use a variable drum rhythm to excite, then calm, irritate and stimulate someone who is ill and induce spasms, contractions, and vibrations which can stimulate the healing ability of the body. A drumbeat can be a powerful tool in inducing higher states of *dhyāna* if it is made synchronous with the inner sounds as will be described. The *tabla* (*duggi*) or Indian drum is capable of creating several different sounds or words (*boles*), with the one produced by friction against the vibrating drum head (*ghe*) being particularly stimulating to the inner rhythms.

Almost everyone is familiar with the sensation of resonating with others in emotions and feelings but generally fail to perceive this resonance as having the nature of vibration. The *tattvas*, as will be discussed, are considered to be vibrational centers for different feelings or frequencies which resonate with the same feeling or frequency coming from someone else. The *tattvas* therefore respond to the particular vibrations projected from other *tattvas*. Their resonating is perceived by the nervous system of the body and translated finally through the brain as particular emotions or feelings.

One example is given with the particular feeling and vibration associated with anger that is much different than the inner feelings and vibrations associated with fear. It is an interesting experience if you have just undergone some very exciting or stimulating moment, such as barely escaping being hit by a speeding car and someone asks you, "How do you feel?" Typically, you may not know, and there is that moment when you search within yourself to find your "feelings" and then attempt to identify them. Another example of this is when you are strangely "moved" by some scent, sound, color, or scene and you again have the problems of inner searching in an attempt to identify the feeling. Many times, the inner vibration becomes associated with some memory of a particular event and you identify the feelings or vibrations as being the same. Similarly, you can arouse a particular feeling using a particular memory or mental image.

With this brief introduction, Table 1 in *Part E* should be consulted to follow the remainder of this chapter. Each of the four levels of the Self can be ascribed to having attributes, characteristics, natures, or individual traits which are contained within elements called *tattvas* that distinguish the individual at a particular level of the ascension from the Pre-Spirit to the gross manifested form. These elements allow the interaction or coupling between the subtle and physical aspects of the Self as well as serving to define the individual characteristics of the Self, and hence they constitute an interlocking system which completely defines what you are and how you can function at each level. In other words, your basic individual characteristics must be manifested in your reactions to the outside world and must also be controllable to some degree. Since these elements define the pieces that constitute your individuality, it is essential to understand them and learn to work with them if you are to change yourself or some nature of yourself.

The *tattvas* are considered to be grouped within discrete areas of the body into conglomerates called *chakras*. The location of these *chakras* is chosen since it is within these areas that the greatest feelings are found associated with the contained *tattvas*. *Chakras*, like *tattvas*, cannot be directly changed or altered, but rather take on their attributes to support the chosen dedicated effort or game. As an example, you cannot change any of the *tattvas* within the *Svādhishthāna* to make you feel wise and happy when you are sunk into the game of being depressed. Only when you change your dedicated purpose, will the *tattvas* and hence the *chakras* change.

A further consideration of the ancients that is experiential is that the bottom of the body or the sexual region contains the *tattvas* and *chakras* that are the most subtle or non-physical in nature. As the *tattvas* and *chakras* are experienced or activated at higher and higher levels in the body, they become more physical in nature and less subtle until at the throat and forehead they can be readily identified with normal physiological and psychological functions. For instance, at the Soul level the *tattvas* have to do with intention rather than the execution of activities done at the physical level. There is one other *chakra* located at the top or near the top of the head which serves the abstract function of the connection with the higher or Divine powers.

The *chakras* are subtle organs with two functions within the body. The first is to provide evolutionary steps from the unmanifest to the manifested real world, and the second is to interface the subtle forces with the physical forces. As an interface, they are as a radio set or a converter that can receive an unmanifest feeling or product of a thought and convert it into a sensation or vice versa. *Chakras* are the instruments which provide physical human beings the ability to experience a continual connection between the manifest and the mystical, subtle, or unseen world. The forefront of studies related to neurotransmitters and neuropeptides suggest that the activity of these molecules may serve as the radio receiver coupling the unmanifest thoughts and feelings with physical responses within the body. The sites of activation or generation of these molecules may well correspond to the regions cited by the ancients for the location of the *chakras* and *tattvas*. Since modern science is still unable to define the exact location or functions of this physiological interaction we will remain with the ancient system of classification since it is agreeable with experience and application.

The *Mulādhāra chakra* is the root support for all of the others and is generally described as having a characteristic of the earth as the source of all materials and life itself. This *chakra* is the subtlest of them all and determines or sets the basic characteristic of your life. It is, for instance, the *chakra* that determines whether your world or day is going to be bright with everything going your way or the world of gloom and failure with everything going wrong. This basic nature of your world is related to smell, and you can readily understand how you can speak of the odor or smell as being sweet and stimulating or distasteful and bitter. This *chakra* has four *tattvas* associated with it which firstly define the identity, separation, and relationship of "I," "This," and "That." This definition is considered as the first materialization of the concept of "I" which is a projection of the Divine nature consisting of two separate natures: the masculine as *Shiva* and the feminine as *Shakti* or of the potential and manifest forces. Both of these fundamental forces shape how the "I," "This," and "That" are to be experienced.

One encounters variations of this interpretation sometimes in a nightmare or a high fever when the distinction between these three can be very blurred. The *Mulādhāra chakra* also contains the *tattva* of *māyā* which is the first step toward the creation of a manifested Self. This *tattva* serves the main function of eliminating all of the possible worlds and natures that the manifested Self could take and limits it to some relatively narrow possibility. It is at this stage that prior existences can start to shape who or what we are or the very basic urges that arise from the Divine or eternal form. The *Mulādhāra chakra* is also compared to the feet of the body in as much as they maintain a "grounding" as well as set a direction of move-ment.

The *Svādhishthāna chakra* is the next *chakra* lying in the lower abdominal area with the maximum sensitivity being at the level of the upper front portion of the pubic bone. The name of the *chakra* means "where one stands" which is meaningful when you are filled with the uprising flow of creative energy. The power of this *chakra* is related to that of taste which is considered more definitive than smell. The word *rasa* for taste has a broader meaning with different characteristics from its usage in the West and include such things as love, bravery, disgust, anger, mirth, terror, pity, wonder, peace, and fondness. This attribute of taste is expressed by six formational *tattvas* located in the *chakra* than when combined can describe your basic underlying capabilities such as: Can you fly? Are you creative? Are you persistent?

One *tattva* or the human characteristic commonly referred to by religions is the *tattva* "*vidya.*" *Vidya* is commonly referred to in religious discussions in the negative form of *avidya. Avidya* is, however, normally translated as "ignorance" rather than the literal and proper usage in *Tantra* meaning "false knowledge" which is quite different from ignorance. Religions refer to this indwelling "ignorance" [sic] in mankind to enforce the need for their counter force of "pure knowledge." This *tattva* shapes your concept of yourself and world and sets the stage for your whole viewpoint of yourself and the world. It is therefore obvious why religions are most interested in this *tattva*.

Another interesting but ignored *tattva* is *rāga* which means "passion." This *tattva* is limited by the typical Western conditioning and thinking which has a difficult time with understanding, trusting, or accepting passion. This *tattva* becomes active when ecstasy is approached. The *Svādhishthāna chakra* is associated with water as in "living water" or the source of vitality in your actions. The hand that is capable of grasping or repelling, symbolizes this *chakra*.

The next *chakra* lying within the center of the abdomen is called the *Manipura chakra* that means "filling of desire." It is a center of expansion which is penetrated by the Spirit in the same manner that the Divine entered into the *Mulādhāra chakra*. This *chakra* is perceived as being symbolized by fire. This center is the source of feelings spreading throughout the body or the center for "gut feelings." It is the center for ardor or heated emotions and feelings.

The *Manipura chakra* is characterized with "seeing" or the basic appearance, composition, loveliness, grace, character, and nature. Its ten *tattvas* are attributed to the sensory perception and the control behind the organs for interacting with the outer world. These *tattvas* create the mental worlds formulated in dreams or visions before they become manifested in the outer real world. The characteristics of the outer expansion into the worlds of the Soul are symbolized by the anus. This appears as an unusual symbol in the modern West where we attempt to suppress its action and sensitivity.

The *Anāhata chakra* is located in the chest and means the "center of living and breathing." It is symbolized by the element of air that is associated with life as well as space and interaction within that space. Its *tattvas* are equated with the physical sensations of touch such as: warm or cold, softness, hardness, and strength. This *chakra* is very important for the changing of the *tattvas* and the interaction between the Soul and the Self. The Soul has access to this *chakra* and those higher through the gate of *pāyu*. This gate exists to protect the previously configured *tattvas* lower in the body within the Soul and Spirit. If this gate did not exist, you could essentially rewrite yourself back to your beginnings with the emotions of the moment. This gate ensures that through the years of development, there remains a more or less stable and constant inner Soul and Spirit. As you become lost in the desires of the world and lose sight of your spiritual origins, it would be easy to attempt to write your inner Spirit and Soul as being dependent upon the moods of the Self.

The gate can be opened, however, at the Self level with the *upashta tattva* in the chest *chakra*. If it did not exist in the chest *chakra* at the Self level, it would be impossible for anyone to consciously change themselves and you would be indeed locked into the robotic nature of conditioning. You are more familiar with the resistance of this *tattva* as an ache or pressure in your chest with strong desires. This *tattva* controls the *yoni*, *kanda* and *Shiva linga* or the area around the perineum. If for instance you become sufficiently threatened, this *tattva* activates the next *tattva* or the *pāyu* at the Soul level as well as the *yoni* and *kanda* which then allow the body, mind, and Soul to change to adapt to the threat with super strength, knowledge, awareness, or whatever is required. As the threat passes, there is often a remaining feeling of sexual stimulation or excitement.

The *pāyu* normally guards the higher *tattvas* from direct action of the Self and this is the gate. If this gate were not normally closed, you could literally destroy yourself with your conditioned desires for power, mastery, or importance. The *upashta tattva* also controls the connection between the nipples and the *yoni* which allows the bypassing of the normal conditioned controls. This connection can activate the *kanda* and *Shiva linga*. This full process requires intense desire or dedication to change or to reach beyond the Self.

The remaining *tattvas* are concerned with the physical senses and the functioning physical body. The last five *tattvas* are the mystical five elements that are the power or nature behind *aether*, air, fire, water, and earth. Earth is the characteristic of having mass, weight, or basic form. Water is the nature of flow such as time. Fire is the nature of energy in all of its forms or manifestations. Air is the nature of space and separation between objects. *Aether* is the media through which we communicate in all of its variations. The *Anāhata chakra* is indicated by the penis which has the properties of being restless, driving, forceful, and the source of starting a new life.

The next *chakra* is the *Vishuddha* which means "reaching out." This *chakra* is felt with the effort to express yourself. You can find, for instance, a lump in your throat as you find an opposition or fear in speaking out, or a tightening of the throat with an effort to express some thought. This *chakra* is symbolized by *aether* which is the assumed media through which communications are carried. It is related to the mouth since it is concerned with communicating as well as interacting. The functions or attributes of this *chakra* are well understood in our culture.

The *Ājnā chakra* located in the center of the forehead is the center of conscious and mental control such as is well known in the modern Western world. It is this *chakra* that is used in interacting with the outside world and with others without external direction or controls. This *chakra* can be equated with the self-directed and controlled interaction with others and the outer world.

The *Sahasrāra chakra* located at the top of the head is an organ for reaching into the unmanifest in order to enhance the manifested world. This *chakra* is a coupling between the total Self and the Divine or the higher nature of other players in the game of life. It allows the direct coupling of feelings or knowledge. It is experienced under the added stress of reaching deeper and deeper into the oncoming moment. It is also a coupling between parallel worlds such that there can be an overlapping of the Divine with the present activities of this world.

One common experience of a *déjà vu* is a common but limited example of the overlap of two different worlds. It is the center for the interaction of the total Self with the power of the game of life or the directive force behind your evolution. It is the *chakra* that connects you to the kingdom of Heaven, to the *zone* of the athlete, or to your moments of ecstasy when life carries you along without judgement. The upper *chakra* is normally suppressed in the modern adult world where individuals attempt to control themselves.

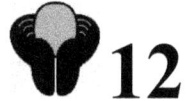

12

KNOWLEDGE, TRUTH, AND THE *WORD*

> "In the beginning was the Word,
> and the Word was with God,
> and the Word was God."
>
> *The Bible*

> "In the beginning was God,
> with whom was the Word,
> and the Word is God."
>
> *The Vedas*

This section will start with a short discussion of the origin of the words "Word" and "Knowledge" which when understood will assist you in approaching "Truth." These words have been distorted over the centuries to hide the hidden power to which they refer.

"The *Word* came unto Abram saying...," this statement in Genesis of the Bible uses the *Word* as the source of the statement and not the statement itself. In Hebrew "word" or *dabar* is derived from the concept of arranging or bringing order into something. Most of the usage of *Word* in the Old Testament of the Bible is with this meaning. In the New Testament, the English *Word* replaces the Greek *Logos* which has its root in the concept of laying something forth. In the opening lines of John and the earlier *Vedas*, as above, the *Word* lays forth, arranges, or creates the world.

In the last few decades, the world has lost a related usage of *Word*. Individuals would give their *Word* about their future actions and the giving of their *Word* was accepted as the existence of those actions. Should an individual not follow through with the actions of their *Word*, they were considered to be less than human or dead to society.

Word was synonymous with a future creation made (to be made) real with the mental creation of the mind called *mantra* and manifested (to be

101

manifested) as *mudrā*. *Word*, therefore, ties the future reality to the present creation of the mind.

Knowledge is the awareness of that which is arranged, set forth, or created by the *Word*. The modern world has hidden the meaning of *Knowledge* by making it synonymous with "wisdom" or "erudition" which means that the source is in the historical past experiences of the physical world rather than an inner mystical source. Wisdom is therefore taken from your past experiences, learning, or thinking, while *Knowledge* is only acquired in the present moment and is instantaneous, complete, and most times beyond personal wisdom. Once *Knowledge* is formulated with the mind it too becomes wisdom and can then be distorted with time and personal biases, etc.

Knowledge is fundamental to the early religions, and in the East it was synonymous with *jnāna* of *Sanskrit* and with *gnosis* of Greek. The common source for *jnāna*, *gnosis*, and *know* is evidenced by the common interchanging of the first letter of "*j*" to "*g*" to "*k*" as was common as words became absorbed into another language.

Knowledge was not only associated with the *Knowing* of the present, but also had to do with the future. Most writers discussing holy people, sages, or prophets speak of them "foretelling" the future; however, many of the original writings considered that these people "created" the future expressed through their *Knowing* of the *Word*, and it was this ability which made their powers so fearful to the populace. This slight shift from "making" the future to "seeing" the future is again the result of diminishing the individual's power and an attempt to make the future rigid and unchangeable. You have experiences of changing the future with "self-fulfilling prophecies" wherein a clear concept or idea appears to fuel its own manifestation. Great people have told of their dreams before they became reality. This manifesting of their dreams, desires, or dedication is that which is described in the *Parātrimshikā* of Chapter Fifteen as resulting from *mantra* or the creation of *True Knowledge*. This is the true power and you as an individual are able to utilize this power.

The usage of the word *Knowledge* in religious writings is the same as the early Greek usage of *gnosis* that was used to define some of the very early Christians as Gnostics. The word *gnosis* was used to mean the instantaneous conception of Truth in its entirety related to some question or search. Truth thus received could in fact be contrary to wisdom or even the past experiences of the receiver. *Gnosis* could be the mysterious insight into reality that superseded the wisdom of that moment. The source of this *gnosis* was related to an indwelling spirit or force similar to that described in the *Parātriṃshikā*. In the modern world, you are taught to desire *Knowledge* [sic] so that it will give you status or polish in society.

A large portion of our society is used to impart this wisdom including the schools, colleges, newspapers, television, books, magazines, advertise-ments, speeches, and conversations. There are, however, all kinds of op-posing forces attempting to discourage the attainment of *gnosis* or *jnāna*. Jesus speaks directly to this in his accusation of church officials as having taken away the keys to *gnosis* despite their mastery of the "biblical law." The Book of Thomas, written even before the Gospels of the New Testament of the Bible dwells on the nature of Truth or *gnosis*. In one passage it states that the church leaders are like the dog in the manger which will not let others eat nor can it eat the hay (truth or *gnosis*).

The early Christians used knowledge (*gnosis*), truth (*alethes*), and word (*logos*) almost synonymously. Each of these words was used to provide a way or opening to freedom or to the kingdom of Heaven. The religions of India used the same words for the same purpose namely: *jnāna*, *satya*, and *vāk*. Truth or *satya* was used in both languages as implying the actual state of reality without being hidden or distorted.

A large proportion of the teachings of the world's religions can be summarized as saying that the *Word, Knowledge,* or *Truth* will make you free. This offered freedom is the release from bondage of something like the Garden of Eden wherein you are only an enslaved dweller conforming to the wishes of the keepers. This, of course, refers to the conditioned civilized world as discussed before, wherein you are a robot or an animal conforming to the rules. You are not much different than Adam and Eve guarding or keeping the Gods' Garden.

You are expected to maintain your family from outside influences and then your neighborhood and to support your place of employment, etc. You are strongly warned against listening to other "truths" (such as that of "serpents"). For instance, you are not to talk about politics, religions, sex, and personal issues with others and learning about these subjects is only allowed under the strict supervision of the priests of the churches or colleges.

Referrals to the Adam and Eve story are generally distorted including the *sin* of Adam. You are supposed to have been born into the world with the sin of Adam and that sin is taught to be that of having listened to Eve who listened to the serpent. Contrary to the institutional interpretation, the *original sin* of Adam and Eve was the bondage in the Garden of Eden, and you are today reborn into the same enslaved state or sin. You, like Adam and Eve, must find the *Knowledge* that will free you and allow you to evolve into becoming as a god. This knowledge begins with the teaching of the serpent in that you will not die if you find *Knowledge* and seek freedom.

The steps described in the story of the Garden of Eden can be summarized as:

1. You must master the World of Law.
2. In mastering the Law, you find that you are in bondage to the Law.
3. In questioning the Law, you encounter a higher power.
4. The higher power provides the access to Truth.
5. The Truth allows the entrance into a higher world.

It should be noted at this time that religions in general would agree with the above summary with one strong stipulation, that "they" are the source of the higher power and control it. A closer look at *Knowledge*, in terms of this problem, is required.

The modern West has a great deal of difficulty with the term *Knowledge* as well as *Truth* and certainly the *Word*, and is unable to equate the three together, much less understand that what they imply is the route to enlightenment, freedom or the kingdom of Heaven of the Bible. The Book of John gives a direct indication as to the meaning of the *Word* if it is read in terms of the creation story in the Book of Genesis.

Genesis gives the account of the creation of the world and all of its creatures in Chapter One and then, in Chapter Two, states that this creation preceded any life or creatures on the earth. This type of statement about creation is fairly universal with the basic understanding that before something can become manifest there must first be the *idea* or description of it. The first creation in Genesis is therefore the creation of the *idea* of it before the second creation which made it manifest.

Plato had also described reality as being a duality of both the manifested properties and its underlying *idea* or description that became expressed as the *Logos* or *Word* behind reality. For something to exist, it first requires a *logos, idea, meaning,* or *purpose* before it can become perceived by the physical senses.

The "...one becoming two..." of *The Emerald Tablet* is a description of this same type of creation or of reality. The term *mantra* of the *Parātriṃshikā* is equivalent to the *Word* in this context, in that it is the intentional, internal, mental creation of that which is to be. Plato argued that the manifested reality could never be as clear as the idea of it, but as will be argued, under the right circumstances it can become much more.

What exists in your physical world must first exist or have been created within your mental world. For instance, if you expect the day to be a great day, it becomes so. If, however, you see that the day is "going to be one of those bad days," then your whole world is colored so that a pall of darkness lies over it all. Similarly, you may pass by some object every day without seeing it, but if someone points it out to you and describes it, then you see it. You tend to forget how it is impossible for a child to perceive the world the way a mature adult can since so much lies hidden and in darkness with their limited experience and wisdom. Another important aspect of this dual world is that everything in the manifest world must fit together. For example, on a bad day you cannot have one person or one experience appear to be joyful in the midst of the gloom. Similarly, in a dream everything fits together, even if you have to fabricate something in the middle of the dream to continue.

13

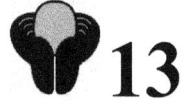

THE SEPARATION
OF THE SUN AND MOON

"Only with the greatest care,
is the physical separated from the subtle
or the subtle from the physical."

The Emerald Tablet

A world that can be experienced must consist of both substance and concept and these two are a dyad, which together define that reality. However, in the midst of the active world, substance and concept are so merged together that only with great care can one be perceived without the other. As an example, listen to the sound of an automobile passing by, can you hear the sound as independent of an automobile? Can you look at a billboard with writing or at this printed sentence without reading the message? Science was created primarily for separating substance from concept. Science, itself, can be seen to consist of substance and concept. The substance of science consists of measurement while the concept of science consists of specifying name and function. Science must be used to separate the subtle from the physical and this as *The Emerald Tablet* states can only be done with great care.

Before continuing, a further understanding of substance and concept or of the physical and subtle is required. India uses two terms analogous to the terms of *Moon* and *Sun* to describe the elements of actuality, which are *rūpa* and *nāma*. *Rūpa* refers to the physical, measurable properties of an object or form such as its shape, size, materials, or color, while *nāma* is the name, nature, or description which identifies that form. Reality is based upon *rūpa* that is unchangeable except with tools, paint, time, machines, etc. *Rūpa* includes and is built upon the four basic building blocks: earth, air, fire, and running water (listed within the *Parātrimshikā*.) These elements also correlate directly with the basic building blocks of modern science: mass, length, energy, and time. *Nāma*, however, is subtle, such as the word "cup." Cup is not a rigid or fixed defining term, as for instance, when a cup becomes a vase or pencil holder. An even further departure is given when a cup becomes a sonic-blaster in a child's game.

In all of these cases, however, the *rūpa* or physical characteristics of the cup are unchanged despite the functioning or *nāma* of the cup. Another form of *nāma* is the image that is invoked by someone's name including your own self-image or ego. Religions use the name of a Deity to invoke the image and nature of that Deity much as an icon. The subtle *nāma* can change depending upon moods, etc. which then results in creating different roles and worlds, whereas again your physical *rūpa* remains the unchanging aspect of physical reality.

Aristotle's term of *entelechy* and Leibnitz's term of *monad* correspond closely to the current usage of the Eastern term of *nāma*. The early Western concept of the physical world and its components was that each element as well as the total manifested world contained within itself a definition of itself that was nonmaterial and physically unmanifested. The chief difference between the Western view and the Eastern was that the West approached reality from the physical side and hence argued that each physical item contained within itself its own monad or *soul*.

A cup for instance contains the sense of "cuppiness" which distinguished it from a bowl. Much of the East, on the other hand, argued that what was physically manifest was but a reflection of what was within or that reality was a projection outward from the unmanifest *nāma*. The East would therefore say that the soul had a body, whereas the West would claim that the body had a soul. The modern world has about dropped the concept of *entelechy* or the concept of a defining spiritual aspect since it cannot be measured. For example, the science of psychology once used the term *conation* in contrast to *cognition*. Conation was the subtle mental process that preceded cognition, action, and desire. On the other hand, some of the Eastern groups have about dropped the concept of the physical, arguing that all is spiritual or only a product of the mind.

In the present world it is difficult to remember that *rūpa* is fixed unless mechanically altered, etc. As much as you may try, you cannot change, move or alter *rūpa* with your thinking, desires, incantations, and prayers. For example, you cannot change your height by a fraction of an inch by wishing. *Rūpa* forms the basic physical aspect of objects and things that are used by everyone. There is a consensus among everyone in your world as to this physical aspect, whereas *nāma* can be (and needs to be) different for each individual. Another fixed aspect of reality concerns energy that can change its form but only under rigorous rules as discussed in Chapter Eight. All of the rest of what constitutes personal reality is not fixed, but rather, as will be shown, can be intentionally changed.

The Emerald Tablet cites the difficulty in separating the subtle from the physical or the *nāma* from the *rūpa* or the Sun from the Moon principles. As an example, the use of the word cup above generally retains its *cuppiness* even as a vase or pencil holder, and most adults would have trouble in not seeing *cuppiness* even in the use of the cup as a sonic blaster. It is the perceiving of *nāma* as unchanging and inseparable from *rūpa* that provides much of the rigidity of the adult world. The merging of the manifest and subtle starts in homes and schools where children are taught to *believe* and that the object of their belief is real. For instance, schools teach about foreign countries, which are never visited or observed, yet are accepted as being real. What a child is told must be accepted as being real and manifested.

It is likely that at first a child accepts the enforced realities from the adults in a similar manner as the enforced realities of their imaginary games. In a game, the child can accept and relate to an imaginary world on some distant planet as if it were real, and in their mind, what is the difference between that planet and the teacher telling of elephants in Africa? Similarly, a child accepts the parent's definition of who and what they are and what they must do to "be themselves" in the same vein as playing captain on a spaceship in their games. The difference of course between the game and the real world, is that in the real world, you are not allowed to change roles or the setting of the role. You must awaken each day to the same game format and that is now "real." In time you become unable to fully separate the subtle from the manifest except with the gross properties of objects. Many of your perceptions tend to confuse the physical with the subtle.

Consider the two concepts *success* and *joy*. Success is generally conceived as being physical (*rūpa*) since to many people it can be expressed in a physical quantity such as ten percent more income or an advancement at work. Joy, on the other hand, is considered to be only a mental or abstract state (*nāma*.) In actuality, however, success is *nāma* since it is the mental definition of how close you are to that which is desired. Joy, on the other hand, is very physical being identified with an inner sense of a pleasant glow or vibration and is therefore *rūpa*.

109

In order to create a new role and game, it is essential that the old game becomes disassembled and new *nāmas* adopted or used. For instance, you cannot fully play Spaceship if you cannot change *cuppiness* to *sonic blaster*. Or for another comparison to a child's game, you cannot carry spears from a previous American Indian game into your spaceship game, nor cook your meals on a fire instead of using a "food converter." Of course, it is possible for a very good game player to play at being an American Indian as a ship crew member requiring a game to be played within a game.

Normally, no evidence of an old game can be brought into a new game. Every *nāma* must fit together in any game with no discrepancies. You are familiar with this change in *nāma* during your dreams, when you step into a new world with new people and situations. If you cling to your old world or dream, you cannot enter into the dream. Insomnia is in many ways a problem of not allowing yourself to let go of your normal world and find another.

There is a common problem encountered with *nāmas* and that is during the period of transition between roles or worlds. A good example of this is the parent who returns from work and sees the family members as having *nāmas* similar to those perceived in the people in their workplace, as for instance, being unreasonable, demanding, and threatening. Another example is how an incident perceived as being unfortunate, such as the inability to start your automobile, changes your *nāma* to being helpless and pitiful for the remainder of the day.

The above clinging to a particular image or *nāma* of yourself or others is many times in opposition to the *nāma* you have with your friends and associates. Your perceived *nāma* of yourself is in variance with that in the outer world or you do not see yourself as others see you. This provides for personal suffering as you are unable to fully react to the outer world. This is comparable again to a child who cannot change his role or *nāma* from being superior to the others to fully playing the new role or *nāma* in their game. It is difficult to separate or change the subtle *nāma* (self-image) from the *rūpa* (the physical body and mind).

This common state can be explained as the rigid union between the Sun and Moon. The Sun includes *mantra* or the intentional creative force of the mind while the Moon correlates to the *mudrā* or the role to be played and the world it is to be played in. The normal situation, therefore, is that there is little correlation between the envisioned world to be and the actual outer world and role that is being played. Another serious problem is that the *mantra* is not that which is fully desired, but rather the desired *mantra* mixed in with the mental image and vision of what things are supposed to be according to the social conditioning. This results in the self-controlling ego trap discussed in Chapter Five in which you are unable to see the separation of the Sun and Moon, much less do anything about it.

The process of separating yourself from the rigid mental controls starts with the *sādhanās* of *Yoga* described in Chapter Twenty-two. The chief *sādhanās* for this separation is called *dhyāna* or meditation. *Dhyāna* follows a single-minded concentration, *dhāranā*, on an object, thought, or concept. Then when the object fills the mind to the exclusion of all else, then any attachment is released to the object such that it becomes without any personally assigned *nāma*. All that remains in the mind is a basic identification with the object that includes all possible or potential *nāmas*. The object becomes, therefore, the fulfillment of any possibilities and contains within itself all possible interpretations.

It is the almost infinite power of "being" that overpowers the mind and pulls you deeper into true *dhyāna*. Being exposed to the total *nāma*, the assigned and specific learned *nāmas* are released and the object can then be seen without the conditioned bias and limitation. As meditation is continuously practiced, the attachments to specific conditioned *nāmas* loosens for all objects of the mind and hence explains the value of *dhyāna* in loosening the bond between the inner Sun and Moon. These practices result in the ability to separate the "I" from the conditioned ego and then to begin the process of discrimination rather than judgment.

One of the hardest and perhaps the next most important aspect in separating yourself from your conditioning is the process of renunciation. The major religions all agree that people are in bondage to the "sins" of their fathers and that they must be able to renounce this bondage before they can find a new life and world. One very interesting aspect about people is that happiness can be found in any society from the primitive societies to the most advanced. Similarly, unhappiness is equally distributed and the elements of happiness and unhappiness are equally well known and understood. The Buddha exemplified this universal condition when he pointed out to some of his followers that they were as attached to their begging bowls as the wealthy were to their money. It is the attach-

111

ment that binds you in the chains of self-imposed bondage and this is a basic attribute of humans.

One of the fundamental *sādhanās* in religion is the process of renunciation or of washing yourself free of your past attachments with the assistance of prayer, meditation, introspection, contemplation, increased pleasure or challenges, or in the taking on of a new life. Renunciation cannot be done once and then forgotten, but rather, is an ongoing requirement, particularly when the body and mind become more active, responsive, and powerful. With the new powers, the past attractions can appear even more vivid and real and the efforts to renounce them must likewise increase. This process is called *walking the razor's edge* since it requires the delicate balance of increasing the inner powers (which increases your sensitivity to phenomena) while renouncing the increasing disruptive influences.

In summary, separating the Sun from the Moon requires the recognition of the difference between *nāma* and *rūpa* and then how your conditioning forces *nāma* to become rigid while *rūpa* becomes more desirous and hence variable. The development of the ego creates attachments to imagined attributes of *rūpa* and bondage to a false world. The *rūpa* of the world must be seen for what it is through the *sādhanas* of *Yoga* and the attachments released so that *rūpa* can gain new *nāmas* and relationships to the Self.

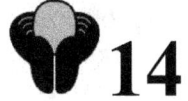

14

THE UNION
OF THE SUN AND MOON

"All of the reality of heaven
can be found to be built on; and becomes manifest
with the subtle union of the Moon and Sun."

"The desired world is made real
thrust forth from the heaven within your heart."

The Parātriṃshikā

This chapter is about creation of a heaven in the outer world using the inner powers lying within your center of being, *hridaya*, or *yoni*. The last chapter spoke of the difficulty in separating the subtle from the physical or the Sun from the Moon elements. Once the elements of *rūpa* and *nāma* are separated they must be reselected and then brought together again much as a stage, actors, props, and script are all brought together to produce a new play. This process can be compared to the imaginary games of children (that have served as a nice model so far) as they integrate their props, themes, and imaginations. However, it is now necessary to add the audience to the children's games and then to get them to participate as fellow players in the game. It would be as if a child were able to expand the imaginary game to include and change the surrounding world including the adults.

You have been conditioned to believe that what you think and believe is reality, and religious institutions have encouraged this inner imaginary game with yourself by giving you the model and goal of you becoming pure in a sinful world. Any notions that there is a difference between your inner world and the outer world keep the Sun and Moon separated. When this separation exists, you have two equally bad reactions, you either blame or credit yourself or the outer world. One of the common axioms that "you must adjust to and then fit into the outer world," is not sufficient. The ancient wisdom requires that you must expand your game to create a perfect outer world that is a true reflection of your perfect inner world. It is not sufficient to imagine or believe that you are changed or different

113

from others. Rather, there must be a complete union of the inner created world of the Sun and the outer manifested world of the Moon. You have occasionally visited this world as described in Chapter Five wherein you are caught up in the activities of the moment and everything became perfect.

Before beginning with further descriptions of the union of the Sun and Moon, it can be useful to consider the problems that are faced in changing a relatively small element in your present life, such as perhaps becoming a more loving person. You may have attended a retreat or course in how to become loving and during the course you could actually start to feel loving, yet a couple of weeks later in the midst of your daily life, you found yourself no more loving of others than before the retreat. At the retreat you were working with other people who were likewise dedicated to finding the loving nature and were willing to follow the instructor. When you returned to work, however, the people around you were not dedicated to being loving nor in perceiving you as any more loving than anyone else.

This problem also arises during the reading of a book about being loving. During the reading of the book, you feel yourself surrounded by the people that the author introduces and you mentally associate with them with the same consequences as above. The problem can be stated as the difference that exists within our mental expectations of the outer world and what the outer world actually is perceived to be. You have definite desires and hopes for what you wish the world and yourself to be and as you attempt to view yourself or the world according to your desires, con-flicts immediately arise. This is like a child attempting to play the role of a schoolteacher as the rest of the children are playing at being farm animals. There is no union of the two games. The reason is simple in that the *nāmas* of the objects of the game are not the same for the would-be schoolteacher and the children playing at being animals. This is the chief problem of most of the self-help manuals and courses in that they may help you to change some of your *nāmas*, but they do not change those used by others in the outside world. It does not help you to become a better person if the outside world does not perceive you as a better person because they will continually interact with you in their perceived view-point of you until your conditioning and theirs forces the continuation of the old shared world.

The problem is that your inner world must be in agreement with the outer world which must also be in agreement with anyone else's whom you wish to interact with. The obtaining of this common world is an aspect of uniting the Sun and Moon. The obtaining of this union starts with *dhyāna* or meditation on the person (or persons) with whom you desire to interact with. *Dhyāna* is used to break free of all of your prior conditioned images or feelings about the other person such that you can react with them in a different role. Similarly, you must in turn allow those you wish to interact with to overpower you, or you must open fully to that which is within them and this is the process of *samādhi*. The starting of the mutual game or interaction can then take place as you both open fully to each other and some goal.

The Heaven resulting from the union of the Sun and Moon requires a deep change within yourself and not the application of a bandage to cover one of your defects. You must do more than a child creating a game with a select group of believing and trusting friends. You must become such a strong character with such game playing skills that others will be overcome and desire to join in some game with you. You have encountered people like this who are described as having magnetic personalities or of being charismatic. They radiate a purpose in life and a power to overcome obstacles. They change the world. You may no doubt sense your built-in conditioning entering in at this point of the book with a fear of such a thing happening to you, or of your inadequacy to do such a thing or your lack of energy and power. It is because of this built-in resistance, that an inner source of power must be found and utilized, as the ancients would have said, "You must imbibe the *soma*," or "You must be filled with the Spirit!"

The change must begin with intensifying the brightness of the Sun. You must find an inner sense of a direction that you desire to follow. This is your dedication that is based upon your inner Will or *ichā*. This is the "desired world" of the *Parātrimshikā* that must be thrust forth from the heart stated at the beginning of this document.

The power of the Sun is increased with the dedication to obtain a new world. The intentional, mental creation of the desired world is called *mantra* and it differs from imagination in that it requires the ultimate union of the inner *mantra* created world (Sun) with the extant outer world (Moon). If the outer world is not considered then at this level of attain-

115

ment, gluttony will be obtained[11] and you sink into your own self-created world.

A good example of the projecting outward of an inner world is given with individuals who are good at controlling animals or children. You have no doubt encountered one of these people when they project their inward world out. Children sense when a teacher "means business" and will not tolerate misbehavior, yet the teacher generally does not directly project this in terms of facial expressions or even in what they may say. Such teachers can only say that they perceive the children as behaving and they do behave. Their inner created world contains well-behaved students and they are able to project this world outward to their students such that their inner and outer worlds are united.

Creating this inner *mantra* or mentally created world requires powers well beyond those used for imagining. In imagining, you attempt to formulate or develop what you desire. For instance, in imagining some desired house, you start with some remembered forms of houses and then modify those concepts to find what feels most pleasing. *Mantra* requires starting with the feelings associated with the final creation and then reaching for the corresponding form. *Mantra* is therefore the first level of the union of the Sun and Moon since the final feelings or physical attributes must be united with the mental imagery.

An example of this is in the creation of a "home." You may have visitors coming to spend some time in your house and you wish to envelop them within a loving home. For most people, this creation of a loving home consists of mental images such as cleanliness and orderliness and perhaps soft lighting and proper music. They have been hardened over the years against anything similar to *samaj*[12] and are now incapable of the basic feelings, of being fully receptive and open to others. There is a vast difference between the intellectual opening to visitors and *samaj* or the surrender of yourself and house fully to the visitors.

If you cannot create this feeling of openness or of *samaj*, you cannot use *mantra* to change your house into a home. You cannot find the union of the inner Sun and Moon, since the Sun is so dim and feeble. The use of *mantra* and feelings in the case of creating a "home" is similar to other

---

[11] See Chapter 7.
[12] See Chapter 6.

applications of *mantra*. Your modern world has suppressed so many basic feelings as already discussed so that any intended world cannot extend much beyond your present world. Your imagination can include a wide variety of potential worlds, but you are not yet ready to make them real because of your conditioned fears and limited concepts of yourself.

A partial and limited example of *mantra* is stepping into a professional role or into a position of authority. Generally, the step is preceded by a learning period under the tutelage of a professional. During the training period, you must learn new material and techniques, but you also learn to take on the role of the tutor. An example of this is afforded by watching your children play a responsible role such as a parent in one of their games. The children are observed to take on the demeanor of their own parents in order to play this part. In some professions, the role must become strong enough to prevent a backslide into one of the old conditioned roles. For instance, a policeman, nurse, or a salesman must be "hardened" against conditioned emotions such as sympathy, fear, or disgust. In general, it takes a long period of time and training as well as some form of internship before one can develop a strong new role.

Some performing artists are good examples of the powers of *mantra*. Actors and musicians can project feelings and emotions in their stage role, while at the same time finding a unity with the audience and react to the feelings within the audience. The projection can be done with words, motion, gestures, rhythm, or music and the development of a changing intensity, all of which constitute forms of a new *nāma* to the audience. The reception of the feelings and emotions from the audience is gained through heightened responses of the body which can be further developed with the ancient practices of *Tantra*.

Almost everyone is trained to fear becoming something other than "yourself." A common fear with students of *mantra* is, "How can I trust what might happen to me if I take on another nature?" This fear generally only arises when the student becomes aware that it really is possible to change the Self. Conditioning accepts the concept of becoming a "better me," but not a "different me." A change requires trust in the future and in a higher power. A basic concept in *mantra* is the willingness to be sacrificed to a higher state of being. This is stated as "dying to the old" in Christianity. You should neither worry about the opinions of others nor take thought of what you might become. Jesus made the statement that you should take no thought for the morrow. The ability to trust the guidance of

117

the Divine can be overcome by inner doubts and conditioned concepts of the Self.

One common problem which limits the power of *mantra* is the rigid concept of what can and cannot be done or achieved. It is easy for someone to say, "Oh, I want to be a college graduate, but I don't have the talents or the time." You are accustomed to take medical advice as supreme law and physiological models as truth. Your culture, however, contains many exceptions to your rigid beliefs, even in the sciences. For instance, there are idiot savants who are considered to be mentally disabled people but nonetheless have talents which defy understanding. For instance, some have been capable of working mathematical problems such as multiplying two six-digit numbers or extracting square roots of a number faster than a calculator. These people didn't know that it was impossible to have such talents. When asked how they found a square root for instance, they replied something like, they just felt what it should be.

People have cured themselves of incurable diseases and created answers to problems that required wisdom which they were not exposed to. Religions also cite many miraculous changes that follow after some mystical experience which suddenly changes a life. It is our tight clinging to what we can't do which limits what we can become. The more logical approach is for you to assume responsibility for your Self and become that which is dreamed of or yearned for with *mantra* and *mudrā* rather than that which you are supposed to be.

If the *mudrā* or role you are playing in the outer world and the world you are playing it in, is not exactly the same as your inner *mantra* or vision, then you cannot enter into the higher realm and you suffer. Your inner *mantra* must become perfect and your *mudrā* must perfectly reflect that perfection. Similarly, as the outer play progresses, the inner *mantra* must also be a perfect reflection of the outer *mudrā*.

The first step of developing *mantra* is that of yearning for a world beyond the immediate. This becomes the first step in change. It is the beginning of consciousness and of independent life. Without a deep yearning, man could be no more than a vegetable or a programmed animal such as in the Garden of Eden where Adam and Eve were initially only obedient pets to the Gods. Until they found yearning, they could not live. The great men in history all reported a deep yearning which drove them on to changing the face of the earth and mankind.

Yearning is considered to be that state of mind which reaches beyond the immediate moment to a world or Self which is but dimly seen such as yearning for mastery of life, or yearning for love or union. Yearning can never be described in detail or touched since it must always be beyond the reachable. Yearning is beyond desire and cannot be satisfied. As you approach it, it intensifies so that the drive is ever increasing. Yearning adds a purpose beyond our daily tasks or the things we do that are necessary for survival.

Life begins with yearning to take a breath, to nurse, and to be comforted. Yearning can be considered as a Divine force and a coupling to the eternal and may sometimes be related to what we call lady luck, fate, or whatever force exists to guide us or enhance that which we are strongly dedicated to do. Yearning is not available on intentional or conscious immediate demand and is absent from momentary desire for immediate results. The Book of Psalms in the Bible states that man can set his direction through life, but God determines the steps. Yearning is therefore the means of initiating the direction to be taken through life or the goals of life.

There is an important distinction that must be made and that is the difference between desire and that which is yearned for. When you desire, you cling to some desired result that can be described and hence belongs in your normal conditioned world and which also is related to the very near future. Yearning, however, implies a direction that you wish to travel or something that is to be found. Yearning does not have a result that can be described since it is always beyond what you can be experiencing at the moment.

As an example, many individuals come into this world with a yearning to master it or to fully explore it, yet they have no image of what that might mean. It is, however, this yearning which can drive these individuals through many confrontations and traumas of life. If you can touch your basic yearning in life, you are probably also well aware that you are traveling quite rapidly toward it. On the other hand, you are also aware of the lack of finding what is desired or that what is desired turns out to be all wrong.

Yearning is the driving force behind evolution and is the chief characteristic of the Sun and it must be united with the Moon and its ability to form, maintain and energize reality.

119

▼15

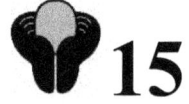

PREPARING FOR CHANGE
The Parātriṃshikā

It is now time to approach the ancient teachings of the *Parātriṃshikā*. This document describes the steps to be taken from this point on. The preceding chapters have essentially given you the preparation or the wisdom that was assumed to be known by one who could understand the *Parātriṃshikā*.

The transliterated letters of the original *Sanskrit* verses are given in capital bold letters. The immediately following text in quotes is close to the literal translation and below it in brackets are pertinent chapter(s) in this book for further reference. Following this is a commentary that bridges the preceding text, the literal translation and the following part of the book that describes the attributes of the higher world that can be obtained.

ANUTTARAM KATHAM DEVA

SADYAH KAULIKASIDDHIDAM /

YENA VIJNĀTAMĀTRENA KHECARĪ SAMATĀM

VRAJET ETAD GUHYAM MAHĀGUHYAM

KATHAYASVA MAMA PRABHO //1

"*Devi* asks *Deva*; how can *Tantrik* powers quickly open the kingdom of Heaven with the knowledge of *mātrena* that opens the path to heaven? Tell me of this hidden aspect of myself which shines forth largely unhidden." //1

[Chapter 6]

This opening statement connects *mātrena* (union of Sun and Moon) with the outer kingdom of Heaven and notes the radiance that shines forth during this process. This phrase can remind you of the statement in the Sermon on the Mount of Jesus of letting your light shine forth which evidences the power of the inner Father (Sun).

121

Devī is one of the inner voices of your mind which questions and is described as the voice of a Lady, whereas the inner answer is from another hidden inner voice listed as the *Deva* or the masculine Lord. The *Deva* can be considered as the source of true intuition or knowledge while the *Devī* furnishes the experience of life. *Mātrena* can be considered as being derived from two words: *ma* and *tra* which mean "preparing" and "bringing together." *Mātrena* is using *mantra* and *mudrā* to create and open a world where *mantra* is similar to the old psychological term, *conation*, or the mental creation of your world before it becomes manifested; and *mudrā* means making the creation of *mantra* manifested in the outer physical world. The word *Tantra* (*KAULIKA*) is a regimen of practices as well as a philosophy. The kingdom of Heaven is that world in which you are at oneness with everyone and everything or when you get "caught up" in the world.

HRIDAYA STHĀ TU YĀ SHAKTIH
KAULIKĪ KULANĀYIKĀ /
TAM ME KATHAYA DEVESHA YENA
TRIPTIM LABHĀYAHAM //2

"Tell me *Deva* about that *Tantrik* power that resides in the *hridaya* as the ruling feminine power of the body, (and tell me) in what way can I find fulfillment?" //2

[Chapters 9,11]

The *hridaya* or heart or center of your being is located in the sexual region and its sense of opening gives it a strong feminine characteristic, thus it is labeled as a ruling feminine power.

SHRINU DEVI MAHĀBHĀGE
UTTARASYĀPYANUTTARAM //3

"The illustrious feminine power is the source of great Divine gifts in the kingdom of Heaven."//3

KAULIKO'YAM VIDHIRDEVI MAMA
HRIDVYOMNAVASTHITAH /
KATHAYĀMI SURESHĀNI

SADYAH KAULIKASIDDHIDAM //4

"By maintaining *Tantrik* practices, the desired world is made real, thrust forth from the Heaven within your heart (*hridaya*.) I am revealing to you the powers of the kingdom of Heaven." //4

[Chapter 6]

The real world is differentiated here from the conditioned world and it is this world which is created by your own volition. This statement is opposite to the conditioning that assumes that the outer socially defined world is the real world.

ATHĀDYĀSTITHAYAH SARVE
SVARĀ VINDVAVASĀNAGAH /
TADANTAH KĀLAYOGENA SOMAS
ŪRYAU PRAKĪRTITAU //5

"Now! We begin with: all of the reality of heaven can be found to be built on, and becomes manifest with the subtle union of the Moon and Sun." //5

[Chapters 6,13,14]

PRITHIVYĀDNI TATTVĀNI
PURUSHĀNTĀNI PANCASU /
KRAMĀTKĀDISHU VARGESHU
MAKĀRĀNTESHU SUVRATE //6

"The physical or manifest is in union with the creative force in the evolving world. Evolution proceeds step-by-step from one realm to another, as the letter *Ka* to the letter *Ma*." //6

[Chapters 7,11]

The union is essential for reality and corresponds to the Word (Gnosis or Logos) becoming manifest in the Western explanation. All of reality must have form (rūpa) as well as name or identification (nāma). The evolution from Ka to Ma corresponds to the beginning of the alphabet to halfway in the Sanskrit alphabet (or "A" to "M" in the English alphabet.)

The reader is also assumed to know that the letters correspond to tattvas or centers within the body which, step-by-step, bridge the space between the unmanifest identity and the manifested Self.

The outer world must be the same as the inner or evolving world. You cannot create a new world that is in opposition with the inner evolving world. You must be patient in the evolution of the new world. Once the world is manifested, each change must proceed step-by-step and you must be patient with the steps. Further, this verse implies that you do not control the steps, but rather they are determined by the Sun and Moon or *Shiva* and *Shakti*.

VĀYVAGNI SALILENDRĀNĀM
DHĀRANĀM CATUSHTAYAM /
TADŪRDHVAM SHĀDI VIKHYĀTAM
PURASTĀT BRAHMAPANCAKAM //7

"There are four supporting elements of reality: air, fire, flowing water, and manifested earth. From these there arises a shining forth preceding the developing of the expansive world." //7

[Chapters 11,14]

Air, fire, water, and earth are used as mystical entities with metaphysical properties (as in the later Alchemy and modern physics) and not as the literal names imply. Air corresponds to the mystical properties of space. Fire corresponds to the modern term for energy that is ubiquitous, but with no physical form or characteristic other than its various manifestations as it changes from one form to another. Flowing water corresponds to time, and manifested earth corresponds to the mass or inert properties of an object. The shining forth is as a first or spiritual creation, or that each of the elements has an unmanifested metaphysical nature that will later be used to define, limit, or shape a world.

AMŪLĀ TATKRAMĀJ JNEYĀ
KSHĀNTĀ SRISHTIRUDĀHRITĀ /
SARVESHĀM EVA MANTRĀNĀM
VIDYĀNĀM CA YASHASVINI //8

"Without beginning, they are the steps of bringing forth all that is known, experienced and created. Everything is truly *mantra*, defined with knowledge, and magnificent." //8

[Chapter 12]

The elements are used to make the world manifest and (when) directed by the mental creation, which defines the outer world, the world becomes glorious.

In this world, the beginning is hidden in the past, and every world that is chosen or created out of this world likewise has no beginning, but is ever continuing as discussed earlier. Anything that has the sense of reality (See verse 4 above.) is defined by *mantra* and becomes manifested shining knowledge or divine experience.

IYAM YONIH SAMĀKHYĀTĀ
SARVATANTRESHU SARVADĀ /
CATURDASHAYUTAM BHADRE
TITHĪSHĀNTA SAMANVITAM //9

"This *yoni* is filled with the 'shining forth' of the four illustrious elements in balance with the expansive world."//9

[Chapters 8,6,11]

Yoni refers to a feminine generative organ which is now related to that which shines forth from the four elements of the world, but in a balance between the inner formulated world and feelings with the outer manifested world.

TRITĪYAM BRAHMA SUSHRONI
HRIDAYAM BHAIRAVĀTMANAH /
ETANNĀYOGINĪJĀTO NĀRUDRO
LABHATE SPHUTAM //10

"The third nature of *Brahma* in the *hridayam* between the thighs unites the Soul with the Divine. Those who do not have the

existence as a *yogini* or the state of androgyny, as did the god *Rudra*, cannot break forth."//10

[Chapters 9,11]

This verse is to introduce a startling relationship of the reader to the third nature of *Brahman* or the *yoni* between the thighs. Historically, *Brahman* has both female and masculine characteristics and the union of the two can be considered to be the third nature. The word *yoginī* means a female *yogi*. The god *Rudra* is used extensively in the early *Tantrik* writings to indicate the power obtained through androgyny since the god *Rudra* was depicted physically as half male and half female.

The third nature or the nature of androgyny is best described as super femininity and it begins with the sense of being soft, tender, and open. You are capable of surrendering to outside forces as well as deep feelings. You can then experience *samaj*. With this force, you yield to flowing with the steps of life rather than attempting to control. You find the rhythm of the flow and then move with it rather than attempting to speed it up or to slow it down. The third nature increases the awareness of the body as will be discussed in *Part C* of *The Golden Triangle*.

The upward flow is felt as very pleasant as well as activating. You find pleasure in movement and in that which you are given to do. Others in your life become more dominant than your own ego and you find yourself overpowered by the feelings of others. You become that which is required. There are considerable references to the *yoni* or female organ in men within *Yoga* writings and it is associated with the *kanda* and *Shiva linga*. This verse ties the previous *hridyam* with the *yoni* or heart to a generative organ.

HRIDAYAM DEVADEVASYA

SADYO YOGAVIMUKTIDUM /

ASYOCCĀRE KRITE SAMYAN

MANTRAMUDRĀGANO MAHĀN //11

"This *hridayam* is the dwelling place of the God of Gods and is the source of union with liberation at the same time. Ascending (beyond) is accomplished with the uniting of the great *mantra* and *mudrā*." //11

[Chapters 9,14]

The lower abdomen being the dwelling place of the God of Gods is taught by most early religious writings yet interpreted much differently to the laymen. The joining of "union" with "liberation" is characteristic of the transcendence to the kingdom of Heaven. The liberation refers to the individual choice of the world to be chosen while the union refers to the intense adherence to the role that is required to be played there.

(The literal translation uses the concept of the issuance (*uccār*) accomplished (*krite*) by the union (*samyan*) of *mantra* and *mudrā*. This "issuance" is through the "opening" cited in the next verse.)

SADYASTANMUKHATĀMETI
SVADEHĀVESHALAKSHANAM /
MUHURTAM SMARATE YASTU
CUMBAKENA ABHIMUDRITAH //12

"At the moment of opening, the body moves expressing the union with a continuing expression and enjoyment of sensual and ecstatic up-flowing feelings associated with a *mudrā*."//12

The opening or activation of the *yoni* or *hridaya* gives rise to very definitive feelings including body reactions related to having an active pulsating super female organ (both sexes experience this.) Intense feelings are obtainable to support any desired *mudrā* or role.

SA BADHNĀTI TADĀ SARVAM
MANTRAMUDRĀGANAM NARAH /
ATĪTĀNĀGATĀNARTHĀN
PRISTO'SAU KATHAYATYAPI //13

"At that time, one attains the empirical form of the *mantra-mudrā*, which was created in the future and becomes manifest in the present."//13

This verse gives a clue that *mantra* must be performed to change the future. The present extant moment cannot be changed, but by opening to an oncoming new world or role in the future, the change can take place.

PRAHARĀDYADABHIPRETAM
DEVATĀRŪPAM UCCARAN /
SĀKSHĀT PASHYATYASANDIGDHAM
(KRISHTAM RUDRASHAKTIBHIH //14

"The thoughts can be thrust forth in time by the androgynous power of *Rudra* to make a clearly manifest and real spiritual shining form."//14

PRAHARADVAYAMĀTRENA
VYOMASTHO JĀYATE SMARAN /
TRAYENA MĀTARAH SARVĀ
YOGĪSHVARYO MAHĀBALĀH //15

"The thrusting forth of *mantra* and *mudrā* with pure consciousness brings forth complete true knowledge and the higher powers of the *yogi*."//15

VĪRA VĪRESHVARĀH SIDDHĀ
BALAVĀN CHĀKINĪGANAH /
ĀGATYA SAMAYAM DATVĀ
BHAIRAVENA PRACODITĀH //16

"The inner great masculine power directs and sets in motion the coming together of the creative powers."//16

YACCHANTI PARAMĀM SIDDHIM
PHALAM YADVĀ SAMĪHITAM /
ANENA SIDDHĀH SETSYANTI
SĀDHAYANTI CA MANTRINAH //17

"The inner perceptive powerful drive results in the obtaining of *mantra* and the power over the faultless manifest."//17

Firstly, the future is changed using the androgynous powers or the power of the masculine and feminine. The masculine consists of the intense reaching for change, while the feminine shapes and defines that to

128

be made real (true knowledge). True knowledge is the same as *gnosis*, *nāma*, or *word* resulting from *mantra*. Finally, when the goal is seen clearly in the future, it is manifested physically and the power over it is maintained by the drive of the masculine and clarity of *mantra*.

YATKINCID BHAIRAVE TANTRE
SARVAMASMĀT PRASIDDHYATI /
ADRISHTAMANDALO' PYEVAM...//18

"The junction of the two *Tantrik* powers brings forth all of the powers in the form of a flowing unseen creative fluid (*soma*)."//18

[Chapters 9,10]

ADRISHTAMANDALO'PI EVAM YAH
KASHCID VETTI TATTVATAH
SA SIDDHIBHĀGBHAVEN NITYAM
SA YOGĪSA CA DĪKSHITAH //19

"The unseen fertile fluid moves, and thus, with this motion, reality is known, portion of his powers come into their own existence, he is a *yogī* (feminine), he is also initiated."//19

[Chapters 9,10]

The hidden creative fluid is spoken of many places in the old *Yoga* literature and called by many names. It has been called the flow of the *kundalinī* in more recent literature. The resulting portion is that portion that is required to meet the particular challenges at that time. The early Christians called it the inner Holy Spirit. The "initiation"' or *dīksha* corresponds to the taking on of a new life or a dedication.

ANENAJNĀTAMĀTRENA JNĀYATE
SARVASHAKTIBHIH /
SHĀKINĪKULASĀMĀNYO BHAVED
YOGAM VINĀPI HI // 20

"Being blameless and with the knowledge of *mātrena*, knows all of the powers (*shaktis*). Even without the training of *Yoga*, becomes one with the assembly of *shākinīs*." //20

This verse is the reason for the universal nature of mystics throughout the world and time. The awareness of the Self-identity as being other than the conditioned (sinful) self, frees one from the blames of the World of Law. When the power of *mantra* and *mudrā* is found, you then realize the full extent of your powers to create. The object of *Yoga* or other spiritual disciplines is to enable you to arrive at this point in evolution and hence arrival is the fulfillment of *Yoga*. As you discover the true nature of relationships with others (See *Part C*), you find a higher social law and enjoyment as an androgynous evolved person.

AVIDHIJNO VIDHĀNAJNO JĀYATE

YAJANAM PRATI //21

"However, without knowing the rules, he brings forth worship." //21

This is the state of enlightenment or of being in saving Grace. Whatever is needed to be known is known. There is union with the perfected (feminine) beings or the *shākinīs*, and all of the methods of approaching the Divine are known.

KĀLĀGNIM ĀDITAH KRITVĀ MĀYĀNTAM

BRAHMADEHAGAM /

SHIVO VISHVĀDYANANTĀNTAH

PARAM SHAKTITRAYAM MATAM //22

"The manifested world is first begun with *mātrenā*, then shaped with *māyā*. The masculine force pervades the boundless created world with its three mentally created powers of spiritual creation, destruction and maintenance." //22

This verse again gives clues as to how to shape the future world with *māyā*. One starts with the awareness of totality and then removes that which does not belong in the desired world. The process of removal is called *māyā*.

130

TADANTARVARTI YATKINCIT
SHUDDHAMĀRGE VYAVASTHITAM /
ANURVISHUDDHAM ACIRĀT
AISHVARAM JNĀNAM ASHNUTE //23

"The inner continual process of life becomes a pure path for the one who perseveres in the rules. It quickly opens to the knowledge of the inner sovereign powers." //23

TACCODAKAH SHIVOJNEYAH
SARVAJNAH PARAMESHVARAH /
SARVAGO NIRMALAH SVACCHAS TRIPTAH
SVĀYATANAH SHUCIH //24

"Because of the radiant fluid (*soma*) one is a great Soul, knowing the masculine powers of *Shiva* and all things. One is without sin, one's will and exertions become pure and shining." //24

YATHĀ NYAGRODHABĪJASTHAH
SHAKTIRŪPO MAHĀDRUMAH /
TATHĀ HRIDAYABĪJASTHAM
JAGADETACCARĀCARAM //25

"As the great banyan tree is contained within the energy of its seed, so also is the "evolutionary upper kingdom of Heaven" contained as a seed in the *hridaya*." //25

EVAM YO VETTI TATTVENA
TASYA NIRVĀNAGĀMINĪ /
DĪKSHĀ BHAVATYASAMDIGDHĀ
TILĀJYĀHUTIVARJITĀ //26

"Truly, bound with the knowledge of the true state, the reaching for oblivion (*nirvānā*) fades away, dedication comes into existence; doubts, anointings and impressive religious ceremonies are abandoned." //26

KRITAPŪJĀ VIDHI: SAMYAK SMARAN
BĪJAM PRASĪHAYATI //27

"Having made the object of worship manifest and united with
that seed, the goal is reached." //27

ĀDYANTARAHITAM BĪJAM
VIKASAT TITHIMADHYAGAM /
HRITPADMĀNTARGATAM
DHYĀYET SOMĀMSHAM NITYAM ABHYASET //28

"The inner seed bursts forward as the Moon becomes full,
coming forth from the inner lotus of the heart meditation with
soma exerting one's own security." //28

YĀNYĀN KĀMAYATE
KĀMĀSTĀSTĀNCHĪGHRAM AVĀPNUYĀT /
ASMĀT PRATYAKSHATĀM ETI
SARVAJNATVAM NA SAMSHAYAH //29

"Whatever is desired and made a dedication to, becomes reality.
The power of knowing all is not reached for but rather abides
within." //29

EVAM MANTRA PHALĀVĀPTIRITY
ETAD RUDRAYĀMALAM /
ETAD ABHYĀSATAH SIDDHIH
SARVAJNATVAM AVĀPYATE //30

"This manifested *mantra* bursts forth from the combined
masculine and feminine powers to attain all knowledge and
powers." //30

PART C

HEAVEN OR THE PERFECTED REALM

16

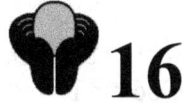

THE GOLDEN TRIANGLE

"By *Tantrik* practices,
the desired world is made real,
thrust forth from the heaven within your heart (*hridaya*)."

"This manifested *mantra* bursts forth from the combined masculine and
feminine powers
to attain all knowledge and powers."

The Parātrimshikā

The Golden Triangle model depicts two possibly perfected states, namely your inner state or source and your outer manifested world. When the inner world is perfected, it is then called the inner Heaven existing within your heart, while the outer perfectly manifested world is called heaven on earth (*anuttara*), or the kingdom of Heaven. The inner world or the inner heaven must be found in order to find the powers to create the outer kingdom of Heaven. Once the kingdom of Heaven is created, then the power must be completely relinquished from the inner Heaven to the outer kingdom of Heaven.

The usage of the word *kingdom* derives from our strong Western patriarchal heritage where the *king* (or heavenly father) was that power that dwelt within you. In contrast to this inner heaven was the outer world which was normally the imperfect world of mammon or the conditioned civilized world. This outer world could, however, be changed to become a heaven on earth or the kingdom of Heaven when the inner power of the king could be projected outward into the world.

As religions became institutionalized and used to stabilize societies, the concepts of the inner and outer heaven changed. As for instance, one of the characteristics of many people in the world of mammon or the civilized modern world is that if they are told of the existence of a higher realm or world, then they will immediately believe that they are in it, if they believe that they are good and follow the laws. If they have doubts about this, then most of them will argue that they will be rewarded this great world after their death because of their wonderful charity or good works in this lower world. The Jews were perhaps the most realistic about this higher realm with their belief that their forefathers had it under the old covenant with God but it was lost later because of the sins and lack of faith of the people. The modern world in general equates their goodness with following laws rather than having faith in something higher than laws (which is comforting when driving at 60 miles per hour on the crowded freeway).

The preceding chapters of the book have dealt with what the inner Heaven is and the heart that contains it. This section of the book will now deal with some of the characteristics that can be found in the outer kingdom of Heaven so that you may use them for guideposts in searching for it. The first signpost is that the kingdom of Heaven is described as a joyful game in which you and others interact in harmony. It is not the acquiring of possessions, power or health and beauty. It can only exist with trust in the game or the Divine guiding hand of the game.

Somewhere in the ancient world some sages described the upper world or the kingdom of Heaven with five Sanskrit words which all began with the letter "M" which became known as the "Five M's of *Tantra*." As a preview to the remainder of this section, the five words are:

1) *Mānsa*: The sensuality of the body when fully coupled to the changing game.

2) *Mudrā*: The expressing of the game or the outer projection of a role.

3) *Matsya*: The vibratory quickening force that energizes the Self and game.

4) *Madya*: Ecstasy as the conscious programmed mind yields to the game.

5) *Maithuna*: Union of the Self, Soul, and Spirit with others and the game.

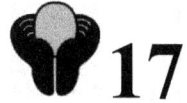

17

INTENSIFYING SENSUALITY, MĀNSA

> "The body moves expressing the union
> with a continuing expression and enjoyment
> of sensual and ecstatic up-flowing feelings
> associated with a *mudrā*."
>
> *The Parātrimshikā*

Mānsa means "flesh" much as in the English usage. *Mānsa* is the flesh of a fruit as well as of the body. It denotes softness, sensuality, and life. Sensuality as used within *Tantra* is recognizing the power of the flesh. Sensuality is allowing your feelings and actions to be controlled by the flesh rather than the conditioned "shoulds" or "should nots" of the brain. The body prefers to move at a pace that feels good and allows the sensing of each aspect of motion, contact, and touch. Sensuality is encountered within the drive for a sexual orgasm when the body tends to control the rate of motion that varies from a rapid rate that jars your teeth to a slow, undulating motion that seems to envelop you and your lover. In interacting with others, a sensual moment becomes the silence, the wild laughter, the locking of the eyes, or just the enjoyment of the richness of the voices. In general, the modern world is well aware of sensuality and little needs to be said about it.

However, the modern world mistrusts sensuality or the power of the flesh. Sensuality is associated with weak character and lack of control. In dealing with other people, sensuality is distrusted as leading to exposure of the inner Self and your own weaknesses. Sensuality is also associated with opening yourself to closer contact with others and their control, which is generally undesired or feared.

As the Western world becomes more concerned with sexual abuse in the home as well as in the marketplace, the sensuality of touching someone else has become highly suspect by the contacting individuals as well as by society as a whole. You are forbidden to enjoy the touch of someone other than a parent or spouse. Being touched by someone else becomes a subject for analysis. For instance, the person being touched can immediately start the judgment process with "What are they after?" or "What do they want?" A touch in the modern culture is generally some form of a subtle command or statement rather than an invitation to a mutual sensual response such as with children.

In the modern U.S. other sensual pleasures are also disappearing. The sensuality of slowly eating and enjoying food is replaced with timetables and more important issues. The sensuality of urinating and defecation is suppressed early in life by learning to take the mind away from such filthy and disgusting acts. A change can be noted in the last 100 years from the sensuality of the anal region to the *tight assed* tension of today. The older literature cites humorous instances of people being "goosed"? When something touched their anus, followed by the extreme behavior shift with their jump and cries.

In today's world, most people walk around with such tension in their anal and sexual region that hemorrhoids, incontinence, and urinating prob-lems replace sensuality. The anti-sensuality forces are imposed during childhood and maintained by the fear of closeness with others or the fear of being judged critically. By suppressing sensuality, one feels that control of the self is maintained and one is protected from others.

The body is easily habituated into becoming only a functional robot. To reverse habituation, a *sensitizing* effort must be maintained which stimulates the body rather than conditioning it to respond less. Some of the senses are stimulated by such programs as art or music "appreciation" classes that, unfortunately, are deemed less and less important in a modern society.

Americans have been criticized by much of the world as being in too much of a hurry to enjoy life, and this is no doubt quite true. To walk sensually requires certainly a slower pace than your normal pace. Instead of throwing your body toward your goal as fast as you can, you can walk and enjoy the side motions as the body swings back and forth. The friction and vibration of motion can be increased until it can be so strong and pleasant that it is difficult to continue to walk. The walking can be made even more sensual with the added sensuality of another person. To walk sensually is a lesson in finding the opposition you have to what others might judge and say about you. You have the same obstacles in speaking, gesturing, breathing, eating, and even in your private daily toilette. It is even more burdensome to thoroughly enjoy the sensuality of someone else. It is a statement about our warped sensuality when we speak of the enjoyment of letting some stranger give us a massage, and then tighten and harden ourselves to our friends and loved ones.

The flesh becomes something that you have and experience in the higher realm, and it is not you. This separation of the identification and the observer is required to fully experience sensuality. The body can become as a lover or an antagonist and as such contributes to the joy or suffering of life. In the normal world, you are familiar perhaps with the body being an antagonist when it is in pain, yet the culture prohibits you from experiencing it as a lover when you feel good. For the body to be a lover, you must respond to the body as a lover and not as only a projection of your own brain and desires. The body has its own preferred sequence of events and timing and these are very important if the lover is to be courted.

Pratyāhāra[13] is the tool for increasing the pleasure of the flesh and requires the continual increasing of its sensitivity. Otherwise, the body adapts or becomes habituated to it and thereby becomes deadened. To be sensual requires the continual expenditure of energy, dedication, and the ignoring of the opposing conditioned forces. This requirement can be compared with the finding of sensuality in sexual play, where the increasing desire for sexual relief increases the response of the body leading to the *vimarsha* of the flesh. Another experience with the *vimarsha* of the flesh is with eating food. You can find a continual pleasure in eating some food or find that the pleasure diminishes after the first few bites, depending upon the intensity or your immediate dedication. (A desire for food is not sufficient since the first bite generally starts to diminish the desire.)

Sensuality is obtained through pleasure centers of the body such as the sexual organs. The mouth and lips are two lesser but commonly accepted sensitive organs of pleasure. The tongue, anus, neck, breasts, nipples, and skin are also organs of pleasure although generally not fully developed. The *kanda* and *Shiva linga* are virtually unknown by the general public yet have the potential for the greatest level of pleasure of all of the other organs of the body.

---

[13] See Chapter 22.

18

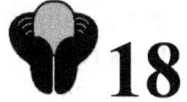

EXPRESSING LIFE THROUGH MUDRĀ

"Whatever is desired and made a dedication to,
becomes reality."

The Parātrimshikā

Y ou have been given powerful means of expression called *mudrās* that literally mean symbols or signs used to open doors or to point the way like a pointing finger. In the past, the word *mudrā* was sometimes used to describe the design on a ruler's ring that was used to imprint a waxen image on a document, thereby giving it the power of the ruler as it was presented to the people. Your *mudrā* is similarly the representation of power, but not the power.

A good example of *mudrā* is a uniform. It is something that you put on that indicates an organization to which you belong and also that you have a delegated power of that organization. The wearing of a uniform for a *mudrā* can be compared with putting on a frown to indicate your inner displeasure or *mantra*. One important consideration of a *mudrā* is that once a *mudrā* is "put on" it has an effect upon the outer world, but it also affects you. To create and fully utilize *mudrā* you must have evolved to the extent that you are able to separate the Sun from the Moon or the *nāma* from the *rūpa* or the *mantra* from the *mudrā*. If this has not been done, then you react as if the *mudrā* is you and not separate from you. As an example, instead of putting on a frown as above to indicate displeasure, there is no separation between the displeasure, yourself, and the frown. If this were not so, then you would be acting and not "being yourself." It is this limitation in being yourself that needs to be set aside before attempting to step into a *mudrā* within the kingdom of Heaven or the game of life or of *Līlā*.

A controlled *mudrā* allows you to enhance "yourself" to become much more than your conditioned self. There are two types of *mudrā*, intentional and those that are conditioned responses. An intentional *mudrā* as used in *The Golden Triangle* is the manifested result of *mantra* or of some directed mental or physical effort. A *mudrā* is more than a uniform in that it conveys intelligence and a coupling to others. A *mudrā* is something that others react with as well as against and similarly also reacts with you to further enhance the intention. You must trust the *mudrā* and allow it to add to your projected world.

Mudrās are used in communicating or conveying concepts, feelings, reactions and roles, from our Self to others. *Mudrās* are your toys that you use in playing and interacting with others. Putting on a *mudrā* changes you as you interact with it. A *mudrā* can be manifested at several levels. The more commonly used level is with the posturing of the body, hands and face, exemplified by a simple smile. A more subtle level is with the inner *spanda* or *tattva* vibrations as you radiate out passion, fervor, or simple anger while your posturing indicates calmness. There is a level of play with *mudrā* that can be used to inspire others to share with you in pursuing some game or experience.

We are all susceptible to the strong *mudrās* of others as we respond to their inner feelings. We may be as confused with the interpretation of their projected feelings as we are of our own. This transference is the result of making direct connections by resonance between *tattvas* of different people. Eastern religions exemplify this when an evolved person "shows" his state of inner mind or feelings to an audience as they sit motionless. Actors and actresses exemplify *mudrās*. Two actors can, for instance, play the same role in the same play at different times. Both can wear the same costumes, use the same words, with the same inflections and the same gestures. However, one becomes and projects the part while the other only acts the part. Dancers and musicians are aware of this state of projection. Eastern dancers are trained to fully feel the character that the dance is portraying so that they can totally project the feelings. And hence expressive Eastern dance is directed toward *mudrā*, while Western dance is primarily directed to depict a process, flow, or action.

There is another form of *mudrā* that is generally not acknowledged or even recognized for what it is although it is often used. This is a verbal *mudrā* without the physical body additions. Conversations generally start with a *mudrā* that is an outward projection of an inner feeling. The best example of this is with a stranger with whom you are wishing to make some contact. You use questions many times to set up a mood or a possible basis for further conversation. Generally, this opening is relatively neutral and used to see if there is a corresponding reaction by the other person. As for example, you may say, "What did you think of the football game last night?" If the response is also neutral, as for example he replies, "Well, I don't get too excited about those games," then you will typically put on another *mudrā* such as being concerned about social reform and ask, "How do you feel about the new Senate bill on welfare?" The response to this question, if not another neutral reply, can then set up a common but initially limited game wherein both of you assume a feeling, position, or projected *mudrā*. This game can then take on a *vimarsha* or crescendo as both people step fully into it. As an example, you both may become very heated about the dangers of a Senate bill or the greatness of it and get carried away defending some position that might not be normally considered.

A more serious side of the spoken *mudrā* is in using it to enhance or reinforce your own inner feelings or *mantra*. Assume that you are in a very depressed mood. In such a mood you will generally add a "flavor" or a "seed" to an introductory statement or question which serves to test the feelings of the other person. For instance, if you say, "It sure is a dreary day," or "The news last night was sure negative," the response from the other person indicates their feelings and their spoken *mudrā* will either tend to reinforce or decrease your own mood. If they appear cheerful, you will rapidly sidle away and speak to another person. However, if they respond indicating an openness for depression, then you increase the power of the spoken *mudrā*, generally by personalizing it.

If you know the people around yourself, you can choose a particular person and inject a *mudrā* that you know they will react to, and then if you are able, you can intensify this mood or feeling with further statements or questions which will further fuel a building *mudrā*. This process is recognized as "pushing someone's buttons" as you use certain expressions, words, or *mudrās* that they will immediately react to. Television newscasters are a good example of this as they alternately get you terrified about some developing international crisis or inject you with pity as they show you a picture of a starving child. Listen to the change in a newscaster's voice as they switch to the death of some local person. For this they get paid very large salaries. Another common experience with the *mudrā* of the voice is with the pitch of the voice. If you speak to someone socially lower than yourself, you lower the pitch of your voice with more exhalation or toward the *tapas* breath as will be discussed.

Mudrās can react inward as well as outward demonstrating the separation from your inner Self and the outer world. You use *mudrā* to communicate between your outer physical Self and your inner Soul. For instance, a method of changing your emotions or feelings was introduced by Frederick Matthias Alexander in the early 1900's who taught that your outer physical posture can determine your inner feelings and emotions. If you stand tall and straight, you feel more in control and positive. In other words, the body can become a *mudrā* that in turn reflects inward to the soul level much as another person's *mudrā* will also be reflected inward. It is this reflection inward that provides a basis for portions of the *Tantrik* systems of worship. If the outer body and brain takes on the *mudrā* of some aspect of the Divine, then that aspect is reflected inward. Parents know that if you can get Junior to act nice and polite, then there is a shift in his total being. The taking of a bath and the putting on of your best clothes to attend a worship service enhances the ability to worship.

If an outer *mudrā* is utilized in an inner dialog, it can in turn enhance the inner emotions or feelings, fears, expectations or viewpoints until you can become an emotional wreck. This can sometimes become obvious as your posture shifts with some inner thought such as with a fearful or a depressive imagined scene. This inner game can become even more deadly if another person is used to further reinforce your own *mudrā*. A common form of this outer exchange is with rumors or "backbiting," which can completely alter everyone's feelings and viewpoints including the starter of the rumor or the original negative statement. The resulting *mudrās* become infectious and dangerous to a group involved with it.

Music, art, and literature can be *mudrā* since they can also project feelings. The power of the spoken or written *mudrā* can be greatly increased when expressed in rhyme or melody such as in poetry or song. A sculpture or painting can likewise express intense feelings, emotions, concepts, or even ideas. Many religions utilize supportive forms of *mudrā* to increase the response of the audience to worship.

A practical example of initiating *mudrā* is when you are faced with doing something you are afraid of, such as walking down a dark, forbidding street at night. One solution is to put on a *mudrā* of bravery such that your shoulders pull back and your stance straightens with a smooth control of the muscles. The *mudrā* may be generated by *mantra* in which the role of being brave is imagined and made real or it can be more quickly obtained by finding the *mudrā* or snapshot which looks like being brave. The other possibility is of course, that you start adopting an outer physical *mudrā* by pulling your shoulders back.

Mudrās are used to assist in mastering roles or in effectuating changes. For instance, beginning *Yoga* uses hand postures called physical *mudrās*, which serve as icons or objects of concentration to assist the immediate demands of the body or mind. Some Christians use the steepling of the hands as an icon to assist in reaching an open receptive state of worship. The use of a hand *mudrā* becomes an excellent practice to bypass the logical judgmental process. Instead of mentally attempting to reach or create a feeling, feelings of the body can either be directly expressed or stimulated with the position of the hand and fingers.

It is not uncommon to find that your body is moving to express some inner feeling before your brain can formulate a phrase to explain it. And it is not uncommon to find that some *mudrā* of the body finishes some of your sentences. In other words, assuming a hand *mudrā* is faster than an inner mental dialogue which takes more time and might also be distracting. Advance practices of *Yoga* use complex body positions coupled with particular breathing and body pressures that are also called *mudrās* because they assist in obtaining supernormal powers found with trauma. The theory is that if the body can assume the physical characteristics found when the body and mind are heavily stimulated that the energy that supplies the powers can be obtained as will be described in Chapter Twenty-three.

Mudrās may reflect the state of the *tattvas* and their activity. As we learn to stimulate our bodies and to play different roles, the *tattvas* must likewise respond. With their response the shape and posture of the body likewise shifts to stimulate or respond to *tattvas*. *Mudrās* may therefore be used to stimulate the *tattvas* to enhance a role or they may be used to enhance the activity of a *tattva* to manifest a new role. Inner churning of the lower abdomen for instance, which also becomes a *mudrā*, directly affects our posture including facial expression, body tensions and voice characteristics.

A large portion of the practices or *sādhanās* consist of forcing the body through *āsanas* and associated exercises into exaggerated postures or *mudrās* such that the body relearns to respond to inner feelings or to experience inner feelings associated with postures. In the advanced practices, *mudrās* are learned that directly alter the chemistry of the body through motion, postures, breathing, and concentration. These also serve to train the body to respond instantly to the demands of the outer world later on.

145

Mudrās can be seen therefore as the outer projection of the inner state of the *tattvas* or of the chosen role resulting from *mantra*. *Mudrā* is sometimes experienced as a radiant force coming from powerful people with increased *shakti*, which stimulates your own *shakti*. You may become aware of the increase in the power of your own *mudrā* after working with the practices of *yoga*. You may notice that many people either like or dislike you instantly. Something is being projected to others which is either attractive or frightening. *Mudrā* requires the dedication of interacting with others and the expenditure of *shakti* to activate your role and the *vimarsha* of the game which is relearned with *Yoga*.

Unfortunately, the modern world has instilled or conditioned you to hide your inner feelings or to suppress any *mudrās* other than your conditioned "being yourself." You are conditioned to project your importance, possessions, and social powers but not your inner Soul, and hence you learn to suppress your *mudrās*. You are conditioned to hide your innermost feelings and to put on the cloak of respectability and success. This cloak is a physical *mudrā* that is at variance from the inner *mantra*. A nurse for instance, uses the professional *mudrā* to identify herself as a professional nurse as well as to hide her inner feelings.

There is a concern which arises with *mudrā* in that you may expect to "read other people's minds" or to open your own thoughts to others. Do not be confused. There is no such thing as direct thought perception. You cannot read someone else's thoughts or mind. This is partly true because thoughts are not the source of feelings or of intelligence. A close observation of your own thoughts should quickly convince you of this. You have sufficient trouble in organizing your own thoughts without the added burden of someone else's chatter. The important capability is to know the feelings of someone else that combines with their memory to produce thoughts. Language is a tool for expressing abstract concepts, but the feelings behind the concepts represent the source. An example of this was provided with one of the early experiments with LSD when a nuclear physicist was asked to explore an abstruse mathematical formula under the influence of the LSD. Under the drug he was able to "feel" and "see" that which the equation was describing and hence could "know" the implications for the first time.

The *mudrā* is a direct subtle projection of *Līlā* and the role that you are playing. If you are not actively playing a role nor following a dedication, then there is no *mudrā*. As you increase the *vimarsha*, then the *mudrā* increases and constantly changes with the game. Actually, you must argue that *mudrā* precedes the outer action or activities since the activities are but a projection of the role to be played from the Soul. If one particular *mudrā* is assumed, it can be increased with the use of *mantra* and *Tantra* as a vehicle for increasing ecstasy as will be discussed later. As you gain understanding of *mudrā*, you will start to discriminate the increasing intensity or *vimarsha* of a truly holy person from the static dead role presented by a would-be holy person. It is this ever-increasing *mudrā* of a holy or evolved person which contributes to the common description of these people as being "mad".[14]

True worship is taking on a new *mudrā* and is generally expressed as opening to a higher power that has the ability to "absorb" and then to overpower the old "Self." The mystical nature of worship is the changing of the Self in order to perceive and experience the perfection and ecstasy of life. The institutional and popular concept of worship is, however, almost the reverse as we seek a change in our physical world to satisfy our desires. In other words, worship has two opposing interpretations: either to change the Self to experience a perfect world or to change the world to satisfy a perfect Self. The latter clings to the conditioned *mudrā* or emblem of the Self and does not seek to change it. The first seeks to destroy the old *mudrā* and create a new. The latter attempts to suppress the *mudrā* and magnify the outer world while the first desires to amplify and project the new *mudrā* and integrate with the world.

---

[14] See Chapter 20 on Ecstasy, *Madya*.

19

QUICKENING, MATSYA

"The inner great masculine power directs and sets in motion the coming together of the creative powers."

The Parātrimshikā

The symbol of the fish, *matsya*, has been used throughout the ancient world as the symbol for the beginning of a new life. There can be no better symbol for a new life or birth than a fish since the early embryo of most mammals looks exactly like a fish and is found in the embryonic waters of the womb.

The ancients surely believed that you began your life as a fish swimming in your mother's inner darkened sea. In India, the God *Vishnu* took on the form of the fish in His first incarnation in the earth covered with water to start life for all creatures. The astrological sign of the fish or Pisces was also used to indicate the fusion of the spirit into the physical world and preceded the opening of spring and birth. The *Tantrik* rituals used the fish as a symbol for the ascent into the state of *anuttara* or the higher realm of consciousness and life. The use of the symbol of the fish as a rebirth into the kingdom of God by the early Christians is no doubt from the same origin.

The use of the fish as a symbol for the higher realms was also excellent because the inner vibration of the belly of the fish was observed to be similar to the intense inner vibration associated with the quivering or pulsation of being fully alive. Again, it can be compared to the quickening of a fetus in the womb as the mother feels the vibration of the "fish" or of a new life. To the early writers it was also suggestive of the deep inner vibrations produced by the practices that increase the inner vitality or quickening. The fish therefore became the symbol both for the rebirth into higher realms as well as the inner quickening vibrations that create the energy to reach those realms. This can also be compared with the teaching of the inner living waters of the Bible and the inner quickening. Both are related to the inner presence of a Holy Ghost or Spirit required for a rebirth or the ascent into the higher realm of the kingdom of Heaven or of God.

To mystics and modern physicists, the physical world is made real or manifest by continuous vibration. All matter is energy in a continuously changing or vibrant state made real by the presence of the mystical element of heat. Similarly, as you become more alive and responsive to the outer and inner worlds with an increase in reality, there is likewise an increase in inner energy manifested in the form of vibrations or *spanda* (which means "to quicken or vibrate like an embryo or fetus"). The advanced practices therefore use the intentional generation and control of the inner vibrations or *spanda* to control and increase your reality.

Friction being a source of vibrations is considered one of the chief stimulants of the life forces. Frictional forces range from the unmanifest to the gross physical. For instance, you face frictional forces as you attempt to awaken from sleep. The necessity to awaken *grates*, *grinds*, and *jolts* you such that it becomes impossible to return to sleep. A *nagging* worry, and an *irritating* memory are examples of friction between conditioning, expectations, and perceived reality. When you are bored your brain attempts to create friction by judging, comparing, desiring, or fearing. This is the friction between the conditioned responses of the outer self or between the conditioning of the Self and the inner dedication of the Soul.

The physiological frictions in the body are well known, such as the friction of sexual intercourse, defecation, urinating, eating, or muscle exertion. These frictions result in perceptual vibrations, *spanda*, or sound.

The more manifest aspects of *spanda* are not normally perceived as vibrations in the Western materialistic societies even though it is customary to use vibrational terms to specify them such as: to shake with fury, to tingle with delight, or to throb with passion. The emotion is considered to be the cause rather than the result of *spanda*. In actuality, one starts with the *spanda*, and then the brain searches to find the conditioned emotion that will fit. This reminds you of a child who is hurt and then looks to an adult to determine whether to laugh, cry or pout. This is the technique used by some actors and actresses when they want to project an emotion. They first become filled with the inner *spanda*, and then let it magnify as they add the desired emotion to it. If you wish to be terrified you must first find the feeling behind being terrified that is *spanda*. It is also *spanda* that makes the emotions contagious. You can feel the vibrations from someone who is laughing or crying and then find some resonance within yourself at some *tattva* level that will build up into fully perceived emotion.

One unmanifested *spanda* is the *nādam* that is commonly called "ringing in the ears" or *tinnitus* in medical terminology. Typically, you hear a particular pitch in one or both ears, yet when you try to determine the pitch, for instance on a piano, it is found that no note or frequency corresponds to the *nādam*. Efforts by medical researchers to locate the source of the sound within the ear have also failed. The *nādam* cannot be said to physically exist, yet it is a basic *spanda* associated with the coupling between the basic "I" consciousness and the pre-Spirit. It can be experienced as the basic force of being. It is first experienced many times at the time of a strong threat against your life, such as a high fever or trauma. In that case it may be so loud that it obscures even the sense of the physical body and brain.

Many *Hathayoga* writings speak of meditation on the *nādam* as the highest form of *dhyāna*. As the *nādam* gains in strength it appears to change its nature from a single sound and pitch to a number of different sounds. For instance, it may sound like a distant choir, orchestra, or a single musical instrument. It is, no doubt, related to reports of hearing the "angelic" choirs of heaven. At intense levels, the *nādam* can be overwhelming as the sound increases to sound like being in the presence of an avalanche, a huge waterfall or a rushing mighty wind. Sometimes the *nādam* can sound as if it is a human voice speaking, yet the words are unintelligible. The *nādam* can also take on the nature of a drum or bell and may be the basis for a diagnosis of mental illness when one "hears bells in the head." Medical science battles *tinnitus* or ringing in the ear, but without great results other than diminishing the basic vital energy. The *nādam* is a basic sound of the quickening energy of *matsya*.

The more subtle or less manifested *spandas* become controllers as we are taught to respond to the laws of society and interactions with others. One of the chief controlling *spandas* in the modern culture is the *spanda* associated with guilt. We are taught to *feel* guilty and people speak of being filled with guilt or remorse. Rather than enjoying this type of *spanda*, we attempt to fight against it by tightening our abdominal muscles and by pulling our shoulders forward to constrict the chest. Our heads are bent forward and shoulders hunched over to further constrict the front of our entire body. Our anus and sexual muscles are tightened to increase the feeling of control over the Self.

All of this can be contrasted to a child playing the villain in a game with everyone shrieking and threatening the child. The child, rather than feeling miserable and tight, feels wonderful and expands further into the villainous role. Similarly, if you master the basics of the *sādhanās*, you can feel the impact upon your whole body as a thought of guilt suddenly is spewed out by the brain. Instead of resisting it, you can learn to let it flow and enjoy the feelings of the *spanda*. With the unrestrained and unblocked upward flow of the *prana* or *shakti*, your brain and body become more invigorated and able to respond as required rather than in a limited and tension-filled, conditioned way. You become quickened and reborn into a new world. An interesting experiment is to sit quietly and then search for the feelings behind crying and laughing for instance. It is the conditioned brain that labels the feeling as an emotion and what you are supposed to do with it.

One of the origins or the interest in vibration or *spanda* in *Tantra* was the intense and unexpected variety and vibrations found during the *yoni* couplings to be described later. As a couple becomes adept and developed with the practice, the progress can be identified with what can be called vibrations. The vibrations become ecstatic and continuous and go beyond the practice even into your daily life or the workplace where they become signposts of the kingdom of Heaven. Table 3 in *Part E* lists some of the *Sanskrit* terms.

20

ECSTASY, MADYA

The English dictionary gives us the Greek roots of the word ecstasy as *ek*, "out" + *stasis*, "place," hence being put out of place. The *Sanskrit* dictionary gives the root of *madya* as *mad* meaning "heavenly bliss, exhilaration and intoxication." Ecstasy and *madya* can therefore be described as losing control of yourself or being under the control of something other than your normal conditioned self. Something has overpowered you and taken over beyond your normal mode of behavior.

All aspects of ecstasy are, in general, suppressed by modern society and many are punished. The strength of the Western world lies in alert and conforming citizens who are first and foremost obedient to the established rules of society. Ecstasy breaks a person free of social constraints because the conditioned mind is quieted and thereby a person in ecstasy is considered dangerous to the stability of a group. As an example, many mind-altering drugs are illegal, and even medical people are limited to the type and amount of mind-altering drugs that may be prescribed. For instance, LSD is not even available to medical researchers, and cannabis or marijuana cannot be used at this time for pain control, even by dying patients. In comparison there are a number of drugs freely prescribed for reducing ecstasy but none for enhancing it; all of these are illegal. (It should be noted that one of the serious problems with both types of drugs is that your world can be contracted to such an extent that *vimarsha* and dedication is lost and the drug controls.)

The majority of the modern religious observances can be described as quiet and sedate without ecstasy, with little or no independent audience activity and tight adherence to social law. This type of highly civilized conduct can be contrasted with the behavior of many of the early Christians who were condemned for their ecstatic meetings, feasts, celebrations, and claims of finding guidance from beyond the laws of man. A limited form of this type of ecstasy can be found today in small religious groups such as the Pentecostal or the Society of Friends (Quakers.) These Christian groups, who allow a form of ecstasy in the congregation, are questioned or feared by the majority of Christians. These two groups remove the power from the leader and transfer it to the individual members of the congregation. In both of these groups, however, the ecstasy is limited because of another imposed law of the group that limits the range of expression and response (imagine a Quaker at a Pentecostal meeting and vice versa.) These groups can be compared again to children at play under the guidelines of the game to be played wherein everyone responds equally to the laws and powers within the game and not to a central socially appointed controlling figure or order.

The physical feelings associated with full ecstasy can only be described with *spanda*[15] and sexual terms since the source is in the groin or loins with a sensation of a strong upward flowing intense sexual-like feelings and vibrations. Saint John of the Cross had to write a lengthy allegorical book to justify his very short poem, *Dark Night of the Soul*, in which he describes the religious experience as a lovers' tryst.

Opposing this mystical experience of ecstasy is the institutional concept of the source of the Divine Spirit as being remote, in the heavens (above). As such it must flow down into man through the top of his head and react there with thoughts rather than feelings. The concept of the Divine force arising up from the sexual region has been declared disgusting, abhorrent and degrading by the majority of institutional and religious leaders. Religious leaders have stated that ecstasy from this source is demonic and evil and subject to condemnation. This abhorrence of ecstasy was further inflamed by rulings of the early churches that the physical body, particularly the sex, was unclean and filled with sin. Many American churches condemn the practice of meditation today and argue that when the brain is quieted Satan and other demonic forces can enter and take over. This statement equates ecstasy therefore to Satanic forces and uses fear to limit the response of their congregations.

In the modern world the sexual orgasm is touted as the highest pleasure of mankind and a large amount of money is spent seeking this pleasure. Americans are encouraged to have regular sexual orgasms and clinics exist everywhere to teach people how to reach greater gratification from orgasms. Sexually active people are easier to control because the orgasm usually makes ecstasy harder to attain and it does diminish the outer social

---

[15] See Chapter 19.

drive for power. (Compare a sexually satiated individual with the individual with "hot pants.")

There are, however, people in the modern world that quite frequently experience a constrained and limited form of ecstasy in the midst of the marketplace. These people are able to allow some tasks in life to over-power them and to carry them off to a world beyond their conditioning. One simple example of this is mastering a routine and repetitive operation on a production or assembly line so that the operation becomes quite automatic. A point can be reached when one lets go of the thought process and simply becomes part of the machine. At this stage, time, discomfort, complaints and worries disappear, and one finds a state of peace and quiet.

A description of how to enter this state of mind is given as getting into the rhythm of the machine or operation. Gamblers can find an addictive form of ecstasy in the repetitive motion of inserting coins into a slot machine, pulling the handle and watching the dials spin around. This ecstasy is enhanced with the expectation of a possible win. In *Tantrik* terms we say that you reach into the oncoming moment with anticipation, *pratyaya*, which is a part of meditation. Observers of these cases might consider that the participants were hypnotized, which is another way of describing the state of being overpowered. The routine assembly line and slot machine can be directly related to some moving meditations. Some Buddhist groups, for instance, use a walking meditation in which the body is forced into an automatic robotic walk so that the mind quiets and the practitioner enters into a timeless peaceful state of simple meditation or *dhyāna*.

One of the characteristics of these types of ecstasy is that a constant amount of energy is required to maintain the ecstasy or else one either falls totally asleep or awakens to the normal world. One form of the effort is in keeping up the right pace or rhythm; the meditator must find the "natural" gait of the walk and adhere to it. However, there is no attempt to increase the energy nor the absorption in the ecstasy since there is a limited amount of energy that can be put into this type of movement or meditation. If for instance the *shakti* was to be increased, then the energy of the action would increase and the walk might become a dance or uncontrolled movement, shaking, etc. Most walking meditations, however, have a built-in limit such as becoming or looking like a peaceful walking Buddha.

The majority of conditioned people are not able to renounce conditioned control of themselves in order to begin to experience increasing ecstasy and cannot identify the state of ecstasy in others. Production managers, for instance, cannot differentiate between workers who are possessed by their machine operation and those who are intentionally concentrating on their work. They are, however, very much aware of the workers' opposition to any changes on the production floor. They cannot understand why workers resist what appear to be very minor changes, but which, in effect, break the rhythm. Change negates the ability to let repetitive operations take over the mind.

The above examples may not be considered to have social or religious value, but are none the less simple states of ecstasy and useful as a beginning *sādhanā* for breaking free of the controlling mind. (This may be one of the sources of the difference between the common sense of the working class and the dogma of the would-be intelligentsia.) Both of the above examples of ecstasy in the marketplace require or manifest little energy and the relative level of ecstasy is normally quite limited.

The above two examples can be used to point in the direction of finding ecstasy. An effort is required to find the ecstatic state. Ecstasy can start with finding a rhythm either outside or within the body. The rhythm may be a regular beat such as a drum or an inner "feeling" or *spanda*. If it is a mechanical rhythm then the associated *spanda* within the body must be found. The body and mind must then respond fully to the *spanda* by allowing it (it cannot be forced) to increase with concentration and meditation on it.

With the meditation or *dhyāna* the rhythm and *spanda* become overpowering and then with *samādhi* you react with the *spanda* and use it to find even more. As a simple beginning example, when you walk, you must find a *spanda* associated with walking that becomes engrossing with increasing wonderful feelings. As *samādhi* is reached, the body ceases to be walking somewhere but rather becomes an expression, fulfillment, as well as a stimulation for even more.

As the *spanda* increases without limit, the body will probably do the unexpected as it may become an animal, engine, or a tree or become possessed by a Goddess, etc. The limits of what it might become are determined again by your overriding dedication and *mantra*. This initial concentration requires far more energy than you would normally expend in either concentrating on walking, on the scenery, on your thoughts, or even on your imagination.

One of the chief difficulties in seeking ecstasy is your distrust of the non-thinking state of the mind. It is assumed that if you are not intentionally conscious and concentrating on something that you cannot function. This is, however, disproved by considering all of the operations that the body does perform without conscious effort, such as driving a car and walking. The thought of letting the body control the walk instead of intentionally directing it is frightening and the thought of the *spanda* controlling the body is even more frightening. Nevertheless, you must learn to rely upon a dedication or a *mantra* of what the limits are, rather than upon the immediate actions. This is the Faith that religions speak of.

Dancing is an easier method of approaching ecstasy than walking because of the externally imposed rhythm. You can allow the rhythm to reach an ever-increasing intensity and add to it by forcing your body into greater and greater responses. Fatigue adds to the surrender by forcing unnecessary muscles to relax which might otherwise present an opposition to the complete physical response of the body to rhythm. Unfortunately, the motivation for dancing is usually not a search for ecstasy. In the first place, you are afraid of allowing a rhythm to overpower you and the second is that you normally dance to please someone else, the opposite sex or a general audience (which cheers in your mind's eye at your great footwork).

One powerful method of reaching into ecstasy is to use an external *mudrā* presented by a statue or icon. Many people can remember using such a *mudrā* to experience ecstasy or the start of it. One of the powers in Christianity lies with the statues of the martyrs, including Jesus. Many Christians, when contemplating a martyr dying for some noble cause, can feel an inward rising *spanda* as they start to identify with that martyr. There is typically a large rush of pleasure as one allows one's Self to take on the *mudrā* of a Saint or God. Some Eastern religious dancers use *mudrā* in combination with a strong rhythm and dance as they take on a role of a Goddess or God. The dancer dons appropriate dress and uses precise gestures and postures, all of which are *mudrā*, in an attempt to break free of the conditioned concept of the Self and take on the new role. As the God or Goddess is felt entering the Self, the dancer must yield and be overpowered to find the full ecstasy.

The nature of ecstasy is determined by the dedication and the energy used in attaining it. Both of these components are difficult for most people to find or put into practice. You may desire to experience the Divine for instance, but your fears may severely limit your ability to allow the energy to increase. Similarly, as the *shakti* increases, your conditioned mind may suppress the whole process due to fear. It can be difficult for new workers to experience the ecstasy of the assembly line as they fight the quieting mind due to fear of losing control.

The degree of ecstasy is strictly limited by the game you are dedicated to playing and typically most people play relatively limited games. There are games, however, wherein you can appear to be "mad" (*madya*) and far removed from the normal civilized world. This state of ecstasy is normally associated with religious or mystical experiences; however, the outer world may declare you mad and desire to put you under a controlling drug.

The higher state of ecstasy is characterized by the ever-increasing demand for energy or *shakti*. Ecstasy is not a static or stable state and can only be maintained by ever-increasing effort to remain there or to continually increase the *vimarsha* of the game. If there is no increasing *vimarsha*, then one remains in the quiet, nihilistic state of the production worker or the walking Zen monk. The greater the ecstasy, the greater the demands upon the supply of *shakti*. A few religious people all around the world know this requirement well as they find themselves drained of energy after a session of "spreading light" or "pulling people into the spirit." The experiences are the same, they become filled with *madya* and lose consciousness of their own mind and body. All that essentially remains of the Self is the dedication to lose yourself even more in the dedicated game.

Ecstasy is found sometimes while working with various practices or *sādhanās* such as finding increasing pleasure in stretching in an *asana* or the upper sweeping *prāna* in a breathing exercise. But more commonly it is found in the advanced practices or *mahāsādhanas*, where it generally starts with the feeling of an ever-increasing pleasure which permeates the body. As this pleasure increases, the body attempts to maintain it as well as feed it with additional *shakti* resulting in the body and mind becoming possessed by the demand for more and more pleasure and effort. As one continues to work with the *mahāsādhanas* the ability to withstand pleasure as well as the strength to push the body further increases. This can be explained as first concentrating (*dhāranā*) on a pleasurable sensation, then letting the pleasure grow with *dhyāna*, and the pleasure overpowering you in *samādhi*. Lastly, both the pleasure and you interact to search for even more in *samyama* and ecstasy.

Ecstasy becomes multiplied when others join with you in *maithuna*. This starts with the playing with others as a child and then losing yourself in some goal with others. These experiences can then lead to an even greater ecstasy when you become united with the Divine in a common dedication such as finding your way to the Truth or to the merger of worlds. This ecstasy can again be further increased when you join with others in what is called worship to find the union of you, the others, the Divine and the Truth.

As you evolve, the ecstasy in each moment can be continually increased, even while you are in the marketplace. The world becomes a reward rather than an ordeal or punishment and each moment opens to new pleasures and experiences. You seek to find and increase pleasure in the unfolding experiences of life. A model of this is to imagine a person dying of old age and wracked with pain being given a respite by being allowed to go back to relive a day which at the time was considered dreary and painful. You can envision that with the sudden awareness of the inner life and awareness that comes with approaching death, she can experience intense ecstasy in doing what might have been a boring job the first time around.

The highest ecstasy is in transcendence to another world in which you find union with the Divine and/or with the perfected nature of loved ones. The description of this union starts with an intense sexual-like feeling as the union is obtained in the flow of *shakti* and *kundalinī*.

21

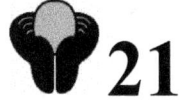

FINDING UNION, MAITHUNA

*"The lower heart is the dwelling place of the God of Gods
and is the source of union with liberation at the same time."*

The Parātriṃshikā

Maithuna or union with someone (real, imaginary, mortal or Divine) can best be explained as starting with *dhyāna* or meditation on them. With *dhyāna* any sense of attachment or control is lost and the other(s) are perceived only within the milieu of the moment and the oncoming moment. When a mutual dedication or game is developed then they become a source of power over you as you step into the state of *samādhi*. Full *maithuna* is then obtained with *samyama* as you and they follow the dictates of the dedicated game or *Līlā*.

Maithuna can be experienced at several levels or intensities. For instance, a simple form of *maithuna* is found in children's imaginary games as has been discussed. At this level children have sufficient union such that they anticipate each other without verbal cues and can allow the play to coordinate all of their actions and feelings. This elementary coupling between the children is no doubt a form of *maithuna* that the ancient primitives had to have in order to hunt and move in concert as they fought together against nature or other tribes to maintain and protect their village. Your ancestors had to be able to communicate at a very basic and holistic level with such things as group strategy or goals, a sense of danger or of success, emotions, apprehensions, purpose and a sense of direction of required effort. Needless to say, the modern industrial world is afraid of this form of interaction. Psychologists, for instance, point to the existence of a seemingly collective mind which exists within a mob which they claim can be very detrimental to the surrounding society and hence a large gathering of people is highly suspect unless it is well organized with the obtaining of proper permits, licensed leaders, etc. The ability of individuals to form a collective mind, purpose, emotion, or action is a simple level of *maithuna*.

As modern children mature, the ability to experience *maithuna* is gradually replaced with judgment and conformance to expectations of others or laws. It may reappear briefly with "first love" as two lovers find that they can respond together at a very basic level, but as conflicts develop, they gradually rely more and more upon conditioned judgments and expectations. Finally, the sources of the basic feelings associated with *maithuna* are turned off with the socially conditioned tensions and desensitization of the lower organs of the body where the source of the higher coupling of *maithuna* lies.

In maturing children, *maithuna* is further diminished by substituting "caring" for *maithuna*. Caring is generally devoid of actual union and consists rather of attempting to control the object of affection or of care. A "caring" person feels superior to the person being cared for and so this is popular as everyone attempts to care for everyone else. Similarly, most attempts to love someone or something are also without union as you attempt to "care" for someone, to possess, to control, to keep from harm, or to make them happy.

Maithuna is beyond love and caring and, in general, may not be perceived as *maithuna* by the casual observer. To refer back to children's games, there is commonly a moment in an imaginary game where two children appear to hate each other or to be fighting with each other as enemies. Another moment they may be busy fighting some imaginary foe with seemingly little love or care for each other. Each child appears to be acting entirely independently of the other children, yet there is a very strong bond between the participants of the game that is the beginning of *maithuna*.

Union in the *maithuna* sense develops only with a common future, goal, and dedication. Civilians marvel at the closeness that develops between soldiers who have had to face common hardships and a common foe. People now pay large sums of money to undergo some wilderness trek with others just to find adventure and *maithuna*. Corporations pay large fees so that their management people can spend a weekend together under adverse conditions in the hopes that they might develop at least some camaraderie. Ironically, in the meantime the government and other institutions are attempting to remove all frustrations from individuals and relationships under the guise of caring for you.

The teenage years are generally miserable as the desire to find a close relationship with someone other than your parents increases. This searching is, however, opposed by conditioned fears of interactions with others as well as the rising power of sexual attraction and feelings. It is at this age that you start to find a delicate equilibrium between the yearning for union with the people around you and powerful opposing forces which keeps them at arm's length. This balance between the two forces generally lasts for the remainder of your lifetime. Adults generally use the sexual force as a means of maintaining a union with a partner, but the sexual union is not that which is yearned for.

The reaching for *maithuna*, closeness, intimacy, or union is called *Samaj* when applied to two people as introduced in Chapter Six. When a group of people seek closeness, it is called *samāj* with a broad *ā*. Neither term is union but rather the reaching for union, or *maithuna*. Both *samaj* and *samāj* have the same basic requirements or characteristics: the yearning for each other, the willingness to be overcome, and the development of conflicts.

As discussed earlier, you are normally kept at a fixed distance from others by the rise of conflicts that prevent *maithuna* with that person. Conflicts can only disappear with a trust in what is to happen next or in that which is dedicated to. In the state of *maithuna*, conflicts cannot exist since they are replaced by the mutual yearning to experience more and more or *vimarsha*. Similarly, only when your trust is in place and *maithuna* exists can you really experience being overwhelmed by the other person.

Yearning is not only mental, but spiritual and physical. The mind feels pleased, stimulated and active. At the Spirit level lies the source of that yearning and an increasing fire and energy. The physical body also responds and the posture, face, tensions and even body motions such as gestures change in an effort to reach closer. There is an increase in the inner energies as the physical body becomes physically more active and alive, and the creative energy opens the Self to a new world. You feel alive and responsive to that force which brings you together. Included with this force of bringing together is the inclusion of all of the past experiences of both people. It is as if there is a merger with not only the immediate moment and the other person, but also with each other's total past and present worlds and roles. As the development of a common dedication increases, there is likewise the sense of sharing the future.

Conflict has two opposing natures: desire and fear. Both of these can become the source of a separating force. Desire, as discussed earlier, is the clinging and reaching for specific things or outcomes. Your general reaction with someone you meet and like is that you desire for them to like you, and it is this desire which is the most common conflict toward finding a union with that person. With this desire you radiate a particular *mudrā* which you have been conditioned to believe is one that others like. Yet as soon as you take on a fixed *mudrā*, you become unable to be changed or overcome by the other person. Most people assume a rigid *mudrā* with people that they know and like which maintains the relationships at a distance.

If you become overcome or united with another person, there must be a change from being the conditioned *mudrā* or self to a new Self. You must absorb something of the other person and become something more, and hence different. The conditioning in your social world has forced you into molds of who and what you are, and these molds are almost unbreakable and bind you to always "be yourself" and to be in complete control of yourself. You have had the experience many times of opening to someone else and then finding that you get carried away with the conversation or interactions until a strong warning affects your body and mind. You find fear in being overpowered or fear that you are changing from your standard self or worse, that you are losing control. This fear of being overpowered is extremely strong and generally you immediately back away and attempt to withdraw or minimize the conversation or interaction.

Maithuna, like ecstasy, requires the expenditure of energy since they both require reaching for more or for continual change. Everyone is well aware of the fact that to join in a party requires the expenditure of an effort to both receive as well as to transmit feelings and actions. A wallflower is aptly named who sits at the edge of a party and does not interact or respond like an inert drawing of a flower. Similarly, in a conversation there must be a desire on the part of all the participants to interact. If one only desires to listen or to talk, there is no conversation. Many cocktail parties seem to operate at the level of passive response in which the rules become, "I will listen to you for five minutes, and then you must listen to me." In many cases this convention further degrades and both talk at the same time.

After the death of a loved one, many people report an interesting observation about their reactions. They found that when they were able to forget that they were supposed to feel a sense of loss, they experienced an added sense of closeness to their loved one. In life, conditioned responses keep people apart, yet after death when these responses drop away, an unopposed closeness will remain. In other words, most people deal with others from a purely conditioned state in which a prescribed manner of responding dominates the relationship. A similar problem results with the sexual responses of couples. It becomes impossible for most couples to discuss sex since they are so conditioned that they must please their partners. Since one partner does not wish to hurt the other, they agree that whatever the other does is absolutely wonderful. With this type of conditioning, couples quickly become locked into routine sex that neither really desires, yet both must state how great their sex life is.

There are a number of popular stories told about the "sinful and obscene" practices of *Tantra* that need to be addressed before continuing. The stories of the practices of *Tantriks* are in many ways similar to the stories told of some of the early *gnostic* Christian groups which were supposedly centered also around sex orgies. The *Tantrik* stories have perhaps received better press coverage because of the claim that they had a perfected (but secret) method of increasing sexual pleasure. (Not true! But a lot of "secrets" are being sold for large sums of money.) There is a considerable wealth of ancient documents available about *Tantra*, whereas the opponents of the early Christian groups perhaps destroyed what documents might have been written about their practices, leaving only the claim that Christians had depraved practices centered around their love feasts (which could have been *Tantrik* in origin.)

In rebuttal to the stories: both the *Tantriks* and *Gnostic* groups were adamantly against sexual intercourse except for procreation. Intercourse with someone without common marriage was even more repugnant. Further, the loss of semen was considered to have been a serious obstacle to evolution even without intercourse. One artifact of the original *Tantrik* rites might be the revered icon of the Hindus, namely, the *Shiva linga* icon. This icon, showing a fleshy protrusion coming forth from a female pudendum, was one of the few artifacts found in the ancient ruins of the Aryans in the early Indus Valley of India. The protrusion varies from a small rounded mound to an upright phallic-like columnar structure. The meaning of this icon has certainly been distorted over the centuries although its use in temple worship is probably universal.

The modern stated meanings of the icon range from the concept that it symbolizes the male and female procreative nature of the God *Shiva*, to the idea that the icon is not a pudendum but rather the outstretched arms of a worshipper with the upper protrusion being the head. This icon is further associated with the formalized beginning of the *Rig Veda* which preceded the other Indian *Vedas* or *Books of Knowledge*. The central theme of the *Rig Veda* concerns the production and powers of *soma*. Also, many of the common writings on *Yoga* describe an inner *Shiva linga* pointing downward from the *Svādhishthāna* that is the base and support for *kundalinī*. The modern Hindu follows an ancient tradition in anointing the Temple *Shiva linga* icon with oils and liquids and rubbing it (*ghatta*). These isolated statements can be pieced together with the *Sanskrit* terms describing the *Tantrik* ritual to reformulate a practice that yields all of the ecstasy, powers and *maithuna* mentioned in the old writings. This ritual will be described in Chapter Twenty-three.

As the physical bodies are brought into close *yoni*-to-*yoni* contact, a *maithuna* results that has the feeling of coupling of the responses, thoughts, and feelings of each of the participants. When this occurs both of the partners respond as one with the same feelings. The bodies and minds find a complete union that far surpasses the union found in sexual coitus. This is further evidenced after separation, as the contact seems to be maintained and is further reflected into the relationships of the outer world.

The highest of couplings is obtained with the Divine when the same sensations are found in the *yoni* as with your partner yet with a more diffuse and penetrating *spanda*. With this intense coupling comes the full opening of the *Sahasrāra* and *Mulādhāra chakras* to your own full potential.

PART D

THE DEVELOPMENTAL TECHNIQUES

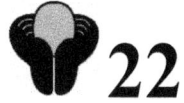

22
THE PRACTICES

C hildren have a basic desire to grow and to master their world as well as an incredible energy that makes it possible. It is this desire and energy coupled with the consistent and patient training of a society that allows them to evolve very quickly.

However, their rate of growth drops rapidly as they start to attain the level of advancement that allows them to take a place in the social structure. This is the result of the gradual loss of the inner energy of evolution and not having a sufficient long-range goal. These two are intertwined in that without a source of creative energy, the ability to envision an evolutionary path is lost, and without the vision, the seeking for more energy is lost. At this stage, the demands of a society and the needs of the body control the individual. The requirements of the conditioned body and mind become dominant and not the inner evolutionary Self or Soul. Typically, with increased discipline in mastering the social world, your evolution levels off and remains at the fourth level as described in Chapter Seven and you go no further.

The largely ignored description of the practices that allow you to evolve further or to regain the energy and dedication of childhood is fairly universal as you look for the underlying structures whether it be Zen, Buddhism, Alchemy, Christianity, *Yoga*, the martial arts, the *Tao*, or Judaism. The following discussion will use primarily the Indian systems since they are commonly recognized to have been the basis for most of the world's spiritual and religious practices. It will be left to the reader to reinterpret the text into the terminology or models of the other systems.

The spiritual or religious practices that can be used for further evolution are called *sādhanās* and are the tools or methods for leading you beyond the fourth level toward finding your own path or a higher dedicated goal in life than that socially impressed upon you. This can also be expressed in religious terms as finding a higher directive Divine power which guides you rather than the conditioning of society. Many people are not aware that *sādhanās* are neither the goal nor even the path toward the higher kingdom since there is a tendency for organizations to sell a particular technique and make it to appear to be something desirable to obtain.

Sādhanās are practices which you can do with your conditioned self and in fact are further conditioning, but they open, energize, sensitize, strengthen or condition aspects of the Self which are necessary for further evolution. Mastering a *sādhanā* has no meaning and you must recognize that it is the step that the *sādhanā* provides that is important. *Sādhanās* are not similar to taking a mood-altering pill, or taking a vacation, and do not do the work for you. Rather than brainwashing or hypnotizing you as some religious leaders argue, *sādhanās* allow you to break free of the brain-washing and hypnotism forced upon you by your society.

Sādhanās do three very important things. The first is to develop discrimination of the difference between conditioned thoughts and the higher, inner, or creative mind. This is accomplished by opening you to the mental state existing behind thoughts. The second important aspect is to increase the inner evolutionary energy. The third very important gain is the development of a faith that there is a higher power within and surrounding you that allows you to reach your major goals in life. It is the attainment of this faith that expedites the evolutionary process and helps to free you from all of the conditioned self-denials, self-imposed limitations, and judgments. This step results in the increased sense of the role to be played and the world it is to be played within. This step amounts to the increase and recognition of a Divine guiding hand or the awareness of your own Divinity.

The result of using *sādhanās* depends upon the goal. Without a goal *sādhanās* can be only a physical or mental exercise. For instance, without a goal of going beyond the conscious mind, meditation results in the relaxing of the body and can be compared with taking a tranquilizer if you are looking for an escape. For most of the *sādhanās*, there are conditioned oppositions that require a stronger goal to carry you beyond the opposition. As an example, your goal of finding sleep must be greater than your desire to stay awake and watch television, your goal of finding a quiet mind in meditation must be greater than the attachment to the arrival of a worry. The success of *sādhanās* depends upon the strength of a goal, dedication, or a yearning.

The following abbreviated discussion will be based upon Patanjali's system of *Yoga*, and more specific details about it can be found in books listed in the Appendix.

The *Yoga* system starts with the *yamas* and *niyamas* that are really the condensation of most of the institutional religious laws. The *yamas* are the laws regarding others and the outer world, while the *niyamas* are concerned with the inner self-controls. *Yamas* include the cultivation of respect and support for others in non-harmful and non-possessive relationships. One must honor others and their stewardship of possessions. One must cultivate the trust for, and follow the hidden power (*Brahmacharya*) behind the outer game of life or an underlying force of goodness which acts as a guiding hand in your life as well as in your world.

Niyamas are the acceptance of the value of the Self as a responsible member of society. One needs to keep the body and mind pure and contented to the extent that one has a positive image of the Self in terms of society. Beyond that, one must develop an inner fire, or fervor of life (*tapas*) which compels one to reach for more in life. As this develops, one also learns to observe the Self as yielding to and fulfilling a purpose in society or life.

Almost everyone in the modern world has been thoroughly conditioned and trained in concentration or *dhāranā*. The modern education system instills at a very early age the necessity to keep the mind upon some task or object. The education system also instills the ability to concentrate upon more than one thought or thing at a time, for instance maintaining a proper stance while reciting, or playing organized games wherein you may need to remember your role while reacting to others and planning ahead. Modern society could not long exist without the ability of its members to control and direct their minds. The highways would be impassable if the drivers could not keep a portion of their minds upon their driving, while listening to the radio or their passengers.

The next level of practices provides the tools for loosening the identification with the body and conditioned brain. As a conditioned, civilized person, you respond to the needs or pains of the body as well as the continual chatter and advice of the brain. The *sādhanā* of *dhyāna* or meditation is used to find the inner needs of the Soul and Spirit. This practice starts with the reduction of tensions within the body which were conditioned within you to force you to respond to the external social world and not to the inner evolutionary forces.

These tensions as has been discussed are the tensions of self-control such as the tightened stomach, anal, sexual, facial and shoulder muscles. The reduction of these inner tensions of conformance to the exterior social demands are accomplished through learning new tensions and postures which become associated with inner forces rather than the outer social forces. As an example, compare an image of the seated Buddha with the posture and tensions of a dynamic car salesman. The seated Buddha does have tensions with his straight back and hand postures, but these tensions are relaxing in that as the concentration upon them increases, the socially imposed tensions relax.

By contrast, a professional salesperson who is "psyched" up to make a sale takes on a set of tensions to make him appear competent, friendly, confident, and successful. His smile, posture, and eye contact are all carefully planned to present a particular image to the outside world that is related to the customer's own socially adopted tensions.

Meditation or *dhyāna* starts with sitting (*āsana*) in a position that has several requirements. The posture generally must be in a vertical sitting position without full back support to minimize the chance of falling asleep. The overall posture must be opposite to the controlled school room "paying attention" posture and instead have the chin and shoulders pulled back, the hands unclasped and the forehead unwrinkled and relaxed. The posture must likewise bring pressure to the perineum or sexual region of the body as well as the buttocks.

The concentration of the mind is upon a single thing that is non-threatening and not mentally stimulating. This serves to keep the mind occupied such that the normal constant judging, thinking, and analyzing activities of the brain are silenced. Typically, you can start with concentrating on the breathing and increasing the pleasures associated with the breathing. As this is done, the body can be deliberately both relaxed and tensed making the back straighter and letting the shoulders pull back, while the facial muscles, arms, anus, etc. are relaxed.

In keeping the body straight, the body is being retaught to selectively tighten and loosen muscles without motion. As this simple *sādhanā* is mastered, the chosen tensions and relaxations of the body can both be increased. In addition, the subliminal tendency to speak is decreased by bringing the tongue to reside against the roof of the mouth. The fingers are held in a fixed posture while the facial muscles, neck muscles, arm and shoulder muscles are further relaxed as the body assumes the traditional meditation pose and breaks away from the conditioned "controlling" or "paying attention" pose.

The object that the mind concentrates upon should be varied as the meditation experience and mastery advance or depending upon your actual requirements (not necessarily what the brain thinks you need). For some people it may be necessary to start with an added visual attention such as staring at a flame or *mandala*. Most people in the modern world, however, have already learned to keep their mind upon some mental subject during their schooling and can start with the inner concentrations. In general, the thing to be concentrated upon is determined by several factors. The first is that it will hold the mind's attention, the second is that it must not be conducive to further thought or analysis.

At this level of selection, you can use nonsensical sounds or words which do not have a stimulating *nāma* or meaning such as a letter, number, or monotonous sound. One very important rule is not to allow the brain to select the thing to be concentrated upon once meditation has begun. Otherwise, the brain will enter in with continual judgment as to how well you are doing or how much better you might be doing with concentrating upon something else.

A common change in the object of meditation about this time is to concentrate upon the space in between thoughts or the source of thoughts. The object at this stage is to experience the intensity of being without thoughts and the powers associated with the Soul or atman level.

With the increase in forced control of the body and the single-minded concentration of the brain, the sound of the inner struggle of the body can be discerned which is first heard as the *nādam*, commonly called *tinnitus* or ringing in the ear. This sound, also called the *pranava mantra*, becomes one of the highest objects to meditate upon. The *nādam* can be concentrated upon allowing the sound to increase and center itself first within the center of the head and then from lower and lower centers in the body until it appears to be generated within the *hridaya* or sexual region.

At this stage, the brain is centered upon the inner functioning of the body, and the conditioned response of the brain is silenced. As time is spent in this space, the outer thoughts and judgments of the brain are perceived as separate and increasingly as unwelcome intrusions upon the central awareness of self. As this meditation is mastered, this separation of your actions and thoughts can be maintained, even as you enter into the marketplace.

In preparation for the outer world or the marketplace, the concentration can be brought to the unfolding moment (but not on the "here and now"). The Chinese *Chan* and the following school of *Zen* taught meditation in part as the expectancy of the unknown. This is exemplified in some of the *Zen* meditation halls as a student faces a blank wall in meditation while the teacher moves around without sound and then suddenly and unexpectedly strikes the student a painful blow on the back. This expectancy of the unknown can be found while reading a horror story late at night when you hear a creak in the floor behind you. This can be compared to the beginning *sādhanā* of bringing fervor (*tapas*) into your life and increasing your awareness of what is about to happen. This aspect of meditation is called *pratyaya* in *yoga*.

Children discover *dhyāna* or meditation in imagined play. The child starts with a desire to play a certain role with other toys or children and then imagines the play and adds sufficient mental control to make the play become a reality. The imagined character given to a doll becomes real. The child in playing learns to project an image, character, action or role into the play. *Dhyāna* is further enhanced with an expectation, *pratyaya*, of something about to happen or of some unknown reaction with the object of *dhāranā*. *Dhyāna* creates a scene as well as the expectation of action. *Dhyāna* is obtained when the object being concentrated upon becomes independent of the concentrating mind and appears to have a mind or nature of its own.

In order to civilize children, society teaches them to conform and to perceive the world and themselves in a fixed and unchanging manner and hence the creation of other realities through *dhyāna* is discouraged or purged out of children. *Dhyāna* is replaced with a societal or family conditioned perspective and exciting possibilities are replaced with more mundane expectations attended by patience and endurance.

Athletes are reintroduced to *dhyāna* by training them to imagine that they will hit or throw a ball to some target without concentrating upon how they will do it. A ball is thrown with the expectation that it will reach its destination and the arrival is perceived as real before the ball is thrown. (The projection of some future occurrence into the present unfolding moment is the basis for a much higher meditation as will be discussed in the next chapter.) The expectation becomes strong and assists in over-riding the conditioned worries or thoughts about the movement or muscle control.

The body is willed or projected with another state that has a power of its own. Similarly, athletes encounter *dhyāna* in finding the *zone* on a playing field in which time slows down and the awareness of the playing field and the players increase such that the athlete finds perfection in perception, thought, and action. A runner's high is a similar state as pain disappears and the endurance of the body is increased.

Religions use *dhyāna* as a method of touching the Divine. As one does *dhyāna* on a Deity for instance, the Deity becomes real and separate from the mind of the worshipper. The *pratyaya* is fired by the longing for or fear of the Divine. When the *pratyaya* becomes greater than normal thoughts, then *dhyāna* and the Divine can become real and manifest. Many therapeutic and self-help systems use forms of *dhyāna* to break free of mental aberrations and pain. Typically, these are sold as autohypnotic or behavior modification techniques. Autohypnotic techniques attempt to introduce an underlying mental view of the Self and world (*mantra*), while behavior modification relies upon changing the physical response and presentation (*mudrā*) of the Self.

The next step in this process is the interaction with the object of *dhāranā* as it becomes independent from your own conscious mind. For instance, when a child manages to make a doll become real, the child wishes to interact with the doll as a separate source of wisdom or action. The stage, when the object of *dhāranā* or the doll becomes sufficiently real and independent is called *dhyāna*, and when the doll is capable of being able to interact with the meditator, it is called *samādhi*. This stage is obviously required for an imagined game to become alive. (It should be noted that this usage of *samādhi* differs from the popular *Yoga* teachings wherein it generally means dissolving into nothingness rather than joining with a creation of *dhyāna*.

175

The final stage in playing the game of life (*Līlā*) is the point at which both the object of *dhyāna* and the meditator or player respond to a power higher than that obtained by either. It is at this stage that the game takes over and controls all of the players (*samyama*).

As you gain skill in making games become alive, then "normal" life can be perceived as simply another game. This normal life can then be enriched and made exciting leading toward actual ecstasy in living. For it to become a game, there must be a trust in some power within the game that guides and controls you. The perception, creation, or acceptance comes as a result of normal meditation. As you gain more trust in this power then it can take on a more definitive nature ranging from a concept of a guiding light to a personal Divine being. Whatever form this power might be conceived as taking, it is called an *Īshvara* or personal god.

This *Īshvara* takes on more and more power as you further yield or comply to its will. In other words, as you reach for perfection with faith in the future or in the *Īshvara*, you are doing *dhyāna*, and the interaction with that created world becomes *samādhi*. This awareness frees (*moksha*) you from identity with the world and you recognize yourself as creator and player within the created world. When this is realized, then you can begin to reshape worlds and roles as does a child when stepping into another imagined game.

The problem many people face is obtaining sufficient energy to play games or to break free of the comfortable role of being "themselves." This problem is overcome with control of the basic biological energy or *prāna* of the body with *prānayāma*. *Prānayāma* begins with two basic breathing exercises. The first is in discovering that you are different depending upon which nostril you breathe through, and that the body will automatically switch breathing back and forth between the nostrils during the day. The second is in discovering the difference between breathing in the upper capacity of the chest or in the lower.

For most people, if you breathe chiefly through the right nostril, you tend to stimulate the left hemisphere of the brain, and the right hemisphere as you breathe through the left nostril. It is no doubt this observed effect which gave rise to the concept of the dual aspect of the body. The left side of the body being controlled by the right hemisphere is feminine, cooling, or of the Moon, whereas the right side of the body and left brain become connected with the masculine, heating, and the Sun.

You can learn to switch your breathing between the nostrils to change your body by starting first with closing off one nostril with a finger. As you observe the effects of this controlled nostril breathing, you can then associate your breath with your mental and physical state. You can then choose a desired state by controlling the nostrils either with a finger or finally with the mind. In general, you will function better in most situations with the equal breathing by both nostrils which can also be controlled mentally.

In starting to discover the effect of breathing in the upper or lower lung capacity it is necessary to first find the neutral or middle point. If you first exhale deeply, the return air flows in without effort until the middle point of the breath is found wherein it then takes effort to bring more air into the lungs. Similarly, if the lungs are first filled with air, the air will flow out without effort as it is released down to the middle point, wherein you must force it out to continue exhaling. The middle point of the lung capacity is called the *vishuvat* that is a quiet center in the middle of effort or change. At the *vishuvat* center, it requires effort to breathe in or to breathe out but no effort to remain at that point.

As you fill the lungs above the neutral point with effort, there is the sensation of gaining control of the moment. This is exemplified by the taking of a deep breath to regain your composure. This is a breath associated with conditioned control such as taught to children to limit their emotional responses.

Emptying the lungs with effort is not taught in modern cultures and is instead considered vulgar and threatening. For instance, if one speaks from the lower half of the lung capacity, the voice assumes a timbre that conveys emotions and power. An individual speaking in anger, lust, fear or other emotions will generally use the lower breath with force. There can be an intense vibration in the voice which in itself carries strong feelings to others. One observation about our modern culture is that the majority of older people have weak lower exhalation muscles and become incapable of deep exhalation below the *vishuvat* center. If you do not run or do sufficiently invigorating exercise that require deep breathing, you lose the lower muscles and the powers associated with it.

One preparatory *sādhanā* called the heating or *tapas* breath is developing control of exhalation of the lower lung capacity in order to increase the energy within the body. This is similar to the runner's second wind in

177

which the air is forced out with effort and the breathing muscles are completely relaxed as air flows back in and fills the lungs up to the neutral point. This breath also heats (*tapas*) the body and can be used in cold weather to keep the body warm. It is this breath that provides a starting point in working with the advanced practices as discussed in the next chapter.

Dhyāna is enhanced by restraining the breath to a narrow band around the *vishuvat* neutral point. The energy can be increased with slight inhalations and exhalation on either side of this *vishuvat* with tight control on the breath such that effort is felt in breathing and a vibration or low sound is heard in the breathing. It is this type of breathing that you use when you're startled such as with a strange sound late at night. When startled, you immediately open the senses to fully comprehend what might be threatening you. Breathing becomes labored about the *vishuvat* which is a combination of holding the breath, but also in breathing intensely with a small amount of air passage. This *sādhanā* provides a base for observing the thoughts and in particular the space in between the thoughts or the *nirvikalpa* state.

Singing or chanting can be very powerful *dhyānas* because they require the controlled forced exhalation, and if done in a group, the uniting of the breath with sound can provide pleasure to the body and quieting of the mind. If *vimarsha* is brought into the group singing or chanting then the words become as a *mantra* allowing the breaking free from the conditioned world and the entrance into a group game of "feeling" and "experiencing" a new world.

The general population knows about *Hatha Yoga*, its *āsanas*, and their value to the health and comfort of the body. There are two principal benefits from the *āsanas*. The first is the stretching to further the motion of the joints, while the second is the obtaining of the awareness of the body. Stretching is known to break up accumulating deposits in the joints that overtime can limit the motion of the joints. Stretching is in itself an exercise of the muscles if the tension is maintained by other opposing muscles.

The movement from one *āsana* to another and then the increasing stretch in the next should be accompanied with the awareness of the motion and the control of the muscles during a slow shift or stretch. This is in contrast with Western exercises during which the muscles are essentially thrown from one position to another, and the important learning of precise control of the muscles is lost. The gaining of the control of the muscles becomes very important in the working with *bandhas* and *mudrās* discussed in the next chapter.

There is another aspect of *āsanas*, however, that is important. This is using the mastery of *āsanas* to increase the power of *mudrās*. As an example, consider that most comedians have the ability to tightly control the posture and motion of their facial and body muscles to increase their ability to express their particular role or feeling. Body language is *mudrā* and it is similar to *āsanas* because it too consists of postures, but postures with a purpose of expression.

As you learn to take on more active and dynamic roles in life, *mudrās* become an added form of expression but they also can be used to increase the inner energy to portray that particular role. As an example, consider the preparation for lifting a heavy object. If you play that role fully, you grimace, grunt, tense your tummy muscles, shift your back, etc. all of which serves to increase the inner *prāna* or bioenergy of the muscles and system.

The flexibility and energy demands of *mudrā* require mastery of the basic *āsanas* and the associated ability or endurance to hold the *āsanas* for a long period of time. This can be further exemplified as the postures taken by the body during intense grief or elation. With grief the body folds inward, whereas in elation the body opens outward. Good speakers use *mudrās* to enhance the feelings they are attempting to project as the body, arms, and face contort. As one progresses into the stronger inner forces associated with *shakti* and *kundalinī*, the *mudrās* become even more contorted and physically demanding.

The *sādhanās* of *Yoga* include some strange requirements for beginners which, although considered necessary, are seldom understood as to why they are required. The first of these are the sitting *āsanas* such as the *padmāsana*. The *padmāsana* stretches the perineum which helps open and stimulate the *yoni* in men and women. A second requirement is for the *uddīyānī* and *jālandhara bandhas* which are to loosen the abdominal tensions and muscles and to tighten the same muscles to force the body fluids (blood initially) upwards.

These two *bandhas* are preparatory for churning. The *uddīyānī* consists of exhaling completely to empty the lungs with perhaps even more exhalation after the first exhalation. When the lungs are empty, the lower abdomen is sucked upward into the chest cavity resulting in an unbelievable empty cavity where the protruding abdomen once was. This upward sucking is accomplished by relaxing the normally tense lower abdominal muscles and then pulling upward with the breath as if you are attempting to breathe through your sex.

The *jālandhara* forces increased blood into the head much as intense anger does except that it is under direct control. The *jālandhara* reverses some of the effect of aging as the blood vessels are expanded in the head countering the normal constriction with age. The lungs are first filled completely and then the lower abdominal muscles are tightened as if in intense anger but with the goal of forcing blood up into the face and head. For this to occur there must be a relaxation of the neck muscles and then the flow of blood can be felt as the face turns red. Both of these *bandhas* must be done with care and gradually extended in force and duration. As mastery is obtained over these two *bandhas* the effects can be obtained with less and less effort and with exhalation or inhalation and used to enhance the feelings in the daily world and hence the intensity of the game.

The intensity of adult games can be increased by regaining some of the child's ability to experience or to feel. As you become civilized, there is a conditioned reduction in the senses as the requirement to concentrate gradually reduces the input from undesired sense organs. If you are looking at something in particular, the field of experienced vision narrows to that object with the other senses attenuated or turned off. As you become locked into particular roles, the perceived sense responses become colored or altered to fit that role. For instance, a garbage collector learns to ignore odors, a cab driver ignores the street sounds, while a mother can turn off the racket of children playing but is able to detect any sounds related to stress of her child. Some *dhyānas* require controlling the senses by turning them off while others require enhanced sensory input.

The increase or decrease in the sensitivity of the senses is called *pratyāhāra* (to restore the senses.) A decrease in the senses is found when the mind is focused upon something more engrossing than the body. An example of this is that you are relatively immune to the pain of stubbing your toe if you are dashing to the aid of a screaming child. However, your senses are enhanced If you hear a strange noise at night which is interpreted as being a possible threat to you and your body. With the threat to your body, you concentrate with *dhāranā* on the sound with *pratyaya* and the breath becomes restrained.

The *sādhanā* called *pratyāhāra* is similar to self-hypnotism, autohypnosis or biofeedback and uses the ability to concentrate, meditate, and obtain *samādhi* to change the body and mind. As an introductory exercise, you can begin with attempting to control the temperature of your hand. If you have a sensitive thermometer, you might place it within your lightly closed hand, although a thermometer is not necessary except to convince your brain that you are changing the temperature.

The process requires concentrating on the hand (or organ to be changed) and then "imagining" that it is changing in the direction you wish. To this is added the use of inner feelings of a flow to or from the object of concentration, and with the hand this can be just an increased flow of blood if the hand is to be heated. You should be able to do this with just a bit of experimenting. Try cooling the left hand and heating the right by imagining that the blood is flowing away from one to the other. After mastery of this you might wish to attempt other controls, such as putting an arm or leg to sleep by mentally withholding the flow of blood or by doing some of the feats reported by martial artists such as locking an arm so that it cannot be bent.

Pratyāhāra in controlling the senses is also instrumental in changing the inner feelings. For instance, you can imagine a fearsome scene and then "allow" your body to feel fear including the inner shudders, tremors, and shaking. In this application of *pratyāhāra*, it is required to first imagine or visualize the scene using *dhāranā* and *dhyāna*. As this art is mastered it becomes difficult to determine which of the *sādhanas* is used first since they seem to become supportive of one another.

Pratyāhāra is also used in some of the advanced practices or *mahāsādhanas* in resensitizing the body. The mind normally is used to desensitize the body as for instance when you learn to sit still in classrooms or as exemplified by some of the ascetic practices of "mortifying' the flesh. One of the needless aspects of aging is the desensitizing of the senses which is further assisted with pain killing or mood-altering drugs. One of the teachings of *Tantra* is, *if you feel, you must therefore exist* which can be compared with the Western Descartes' statement that, *if you think, you must therefore exist.* (Hence the confusion about the possible difference between a human and a computer.)

In summary, the *sādhanās* of Patanjali's *Yoga* or *Asthānga Yoga* are useful tools for the mastery of the social world or of rising to the fourth level in the seven-step evolution model. The *sādhanās* also prepare you for using the higher practices of *mahāsādhanas* to evolve beyond the social world.

23

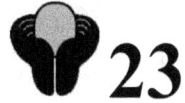

THE GREATER PRACTICES OR MAHĀSĀDHANAS

Mahāsādhanas are advanced practices that can be described as leading toward the accelerated activity of the body and mind associated with the higher realms. As previously described, this accelerated state follows certain traumatic or demanding situations wherein you are able to do supernormal feats or find the state that leads to creativity, *maithuna*, or ecstasy.

There are two basic ways that you can find this higher realm; the first is instantaneous and the second requires considerable prolonged effort. The instantaneous way is of short duration and without long-range effects including the loss of the ability to change at your desire. The instantaneous way also requires a strong outer force that is either traumatic or ecstatic as has been discussed. The important aspect of the instantaneous transcendence, however, is that it clearly points to the higher state of existence and demonstrates the possibility of attaining it under your own volition. This instantaneous route demonstrates the necessity of somehow stepping beyond the conditioned controls of the brain and body. When the transcendence occurs there is always the reported loss of ego, concern, fear, desires, self-importance as well as the attainment of the changes in mind or body that are able to cope with the requirements of the new, higher world.

An excellent example of a practice that leads to the instantaneous route is described in a book written by Jack London, an American author. The book was called *The Star Rover* written about the mystical experiences of a convict who had been constrained with two tightly laced straightjackets a number of times in an Arizona prison. Briefly, the story described how guards would punish inmates by lacing up a convict with extreme tightness using two straightjackets such that the lungs were extremely restricted and normal breathing became impossible. The central figure in London's novel was told by other prisoners that the secret of survival was "to go with" rather than fight the constraints. The hero then found transcendent states of consciousness that he described as stepping back into previous lifetimes.

Perhaps the above story motivated the many seekers of psychic powers (widely reported in the early part of this century) who approached death with extreme methods such as suffocation, hanging, starvation and body restriction. The reasons given were that they wished to find an escape from the limitations of their thoughts and bodies. It can be assumed that those who did in fact find release might have been unable to escape death, while a few of those who did not die wrote about their failures or limited successes.

The early mystery schools were reputed to have used similar methods as perhaps illustrated with the story of Lazarus in the Book of John in the Bible. The approach to death has long been assumed to be a method of stepping into another reality as also related by the glowing stories of ecstasy told by some people as they lay dying in their beds and also by those who report "near death experiences." The modern world appears to be trying to use drugs, visual stimulation from movies and television, as well as loud rhythmic music and sound to traumatize the body, but transcendence of the Self seldom results.

The problem with these systems is that you generally lose a sense of direction or the seeking of transcendence and become locked into the immediate moment under the control of the drug, movie, or rhythm. As a further example, the majority of people who face a traumatic situation without a strong dedication in their life generally "freeze up" or attempt to back away from the situation and will generally suffer psychological or physical damage from the incident.

Another popular technique of seeking transcendence is to use the sexual drive and orgasm to induce such intense pleasure and drive that momentary release can be obtained. As mentioned earlier, with the sex drive, there can be temporary amnesia or you can experience your partner becoming someone else or that you are in an entirely different setting or place.

During these times there is a complete loss of ego and self-importance and the conditioned judgmental brain becomes quiet. The problem with sexual drive is in many ways similar to problems with drugs in that you lose the ability to make changes or to direct the game with a dedicated goal. After an orgasm, you likewise temporarily lose the ability to generate *shakti* and thereby separate yourself further from controlling the transcendent power at least in the near future. You have probably attempted to find ecstasy during masturbation by avoiding an orgasm while maintaining the stimulation, although you also found that this too is unsatisfactory.

Examples of the second route to transcendence requiring long continuous effort are found in some of the early penitentiary inmates who were kept in isolation for long periods of time. Many of these inmates found complete changes in their view of themselves and their world and became contributors to their societies. The isolated penitentiary inmate can of course also be compared to the ascetic who retired from life to seclusion in a cave where mystical experiences were reported. Similarly, many religious figures reported mystical experiences following long periods of isolation and/or intense mental yearning. (The modern penitentiaries are not exemplary for transcendence.)

Another route to transcendence that is more common with spiritual seekers starts with a yearning for the Divine that keeps increasing and finally overrides your normal desires. One approach that has been used at this time is to separate yourself from your normal world and dedicate yourself toward finding the union with the object of the yearning no matter how many days it might take. You might start with normal prayer, contemplation, or meditation and may continue on for many, many hours arousing yourself occasionally to determine your progress.

Typically, your yearning only increases during this period and your mind starts to become confused and bewildered. At this time, you might start flattering and praising to obtain the Divine attention. This period may end after many more hours in further frustration and with the beginning of anger as you then attempt to buy your way with promises of changing your life. At the end of this period, your anger may give way to the sense of being abandoned and unworthy, and you enter into a stage of self-pity as the body sinks into a paroxysm of grief. This intense body response of grief seems as a balm to both mind and body. By this time, days may have passed, certainly more than a day, and you are starting to feel something akin to extreme fatigue and loss of control of body and mind. The yearning, however, has not diminished and usually has intensified such that it becomes overpowering and finally after surrendering any effort of self-control, it seems to totally sweep over you. It is at this stage that you find the union with the Divine and supernatural capabilities.

One more example of a *mahāsādhana* leading to transcendence is that of intense dedication or of self-sacrifice in which you surrender everything to some purpose. This can be exemplified by a soldier on the battlefield giving up his life to save his buddies. It can also be felt by the ancient young maiden giving up her life to the volcano to save the village. In your modern world, self-sacrifice can begin with such things as speaking forcibly with all of your heart at a public gathering or to do something relatively simple like letting down your hair and letting go of "what they will think" as you follow a strong yearning.

The advanced practices or *mahāsādhanas* do not require years of isolation, approaching death, nor body torture and deprivation, but they do require intense effort and dedication. For those who practice *mahāsādhanas*, there is, however, a real danger as stated in the Warning at the beginning of this book.

The preferred method of transcendence taught by the majority of the ancient religious and philosophical writers was to learn to obtain and control intense pleasure or ecstasy. Alcohol and some drugs indicate that this method should work, since the social drugs do in fact reduce the judgmental activity of the brain so that you can find increased enjoyment in the moment. However, when you are under the influence of the drug you lose control and cannot direct the changes, also the use of drugs can decrease the ability to generate the *shakti* during and after taking of the drug.

Because of the universal description of the involvement of the lower abdomen in peak experiences, or trauma, the ancient sages concentrated upon this region of the body and found that many of the results of trauma could be reproduced under individual control. *Mahāsādhanas* are therefore characterized as centering on the lower abdominal or sexual region of the body and the special sexual-like or novel energy responses within the body. There is little doubt that these practices influence the production of hormones and contribute to some large swings in the biochemistry of the body to offer a modern explanation of the effects of both trauma and *mahāsādhanas*. Of special interest, however, is the fact that whatever the mechanism may be, it shifts to meet the needs of the body and the outer world.

The process of breaking free from conditioning requires prolonged effort and dedication and can be described in the ancient terms as separating the Sun and Moon and then recombining them to form a new world or heaven. This can also be described as creating the mental perception of the desired change (*mantra*) after separating the old Sun and Moon union, and then manifesting the change (*mudrā*) with a recombined Sun and Moon.

Chapter Nine discusses the basis for the advanced practices with the description of the androgynous nature and forces as well as the discussion of the suppression of androgyny by society. The starting position of advanced practices is to undo the conditioning of society and this starts with the lower abdomen. For the following *mahāsādhanas*, it is recommended that you should be familiar with and capable of doing the *bandhas* and the ten *mudrās* described in the *Haṭhayogapradīpikā*, which is a basic handbook for *Hatha Yoga*. The following text, however, will give a brief outline of the methods to be used to accomplish these.

WARNING: When *mahāsādhanas* are begun, you should watch very carefully your intake of protein. If you find strange pressures, aches, vibrations in the chest or head, you should quickly attempt to eat some protein. This will generally correct the problem within less than an hour. If you allow your protein to become depleted by stinting on your diet, the *Haṭhayogapradīpikā* says quite correctly that the inner fire will quickly consume the body. It should be constantly noted that a great deal of changing will take place in the body and mind with the *mahāsādhanas* that requires added nutrition. Many people claim to feel like teenagers going through another pubescent change.

After the *uddīyānī* and *jālandhara*, described in the last chapter, are mastered, they can be combined with deep inner muscle movements to develop another set of muscles using the ten *mudrās* of the *Haṭhayogapradīpikā*. These *mudrās* consist of pounding, stretching, pulling, pressing, aligning, churning and tensioning of the lower muscles. It is easy to perceive that this set of practices mimics that tensioning and churning found during a traumatic encounter.

One important developmental exercise of these *mudrās* uses the upper pulling which feels like attempting to suck up water through the perineum (or your sex organ) or to imagine that you are grasping large pearls with an imagined opening to the *yoni* and then pulling them upwards toward the solar plexus.[16] This must be repeated daily until it becomes very pleasurable and forceful. As this exercise is mastered, new controls are found and muscles are developed that are required for churning. There is also another very pleasant and powerful movement that takes place that is generally described as an inner upper flowing of sexual fluids or semen called *ūrdhva retas*. This process is described as *khechari mudrā* or the tenth *mudrā* in which the upper flow from the *yoni* is described as the tongue of *Agni* or fire (*Jihva*) and the route that it takes is called the path of the Sun (*ravechārī.*) The process of inducing this flow follows an inner regular contraction and relaxation that becomes automatic with some effort as will be understood. This total process is also called the processing of *soma* in the *Rig Veda* that is similarly described as pounding, pressing, pulling, churning, etc. It should be noted that sexual orgasm should be avoided, otherwise it will make the *mahāsādhanas* more difficult to do, although an occasional orgasm does no permanent damage contrary to what is stated in the various religious schools. (Sexual intercourse and orgasm can be replaced with a higher and more ecstatic form of union as will be outlined later.)

The *yoni* is further developed by sitting cross-legged in the meditation pose and applying pressure to the *yoni* with a soft compressible material such that the pressure is comfortable but not sufficient to fully support the weight of the body. This is an easy substitute for the *siddhāsana Yoga* pose that adds the direct pressure to the *yoni* with the side of one foot as well as frontal pressure with the other heel that stimulates the base of the *Shiva linga*.

As you concentrate on the *yoni*, the nipples are gently massaged and connections between the nipples and *yoni* are searched for. (The stimulation of the nipples is not generally specified in the ancient writings, although it is certainly understood. For instance, note the ancient naming of the nipples as the Sun and the Moon and the rendition of an ancient drawing of the *kāmakalā* found on the back cover of the book.) With time, a very pleasant sensation can be found in the *yoni* with nipple stimulation (about 50% of men and women start with a slight connection). At this time, the upward lifting of pearls should be added to the nipple stimulation and increased pleasurable sensations sought for.

---

[16] Greek: "nerve center for the Sun"

The breath needs to be brought under control with breath retention called *kumbhaka* developed with practices well described in other manuals. There is another form of breathing that needs to be mastered for added power and enjoyment and that is the limited breathing around the *vishuvat* of the breath as described in the previous chapter. The desired sensations are that of *kumbhaka*, but breathing takes place at a minimal level with very little motion of the lungs about the central point. It is similar to the breathing during the intense listening for some faint threatening noise (*pratyaya*.) This breath increases the flow of *shakti* when combined with churning and the previous practices. This is an ideal breath for reaching for some Divine experience or intense prayer.

There is another valuable breathing exercise and that is using the *tapas* or heating breath combined with *kumbhaka*. This approximates the double straightjacket effect in that the lungs are emptied and then the breath is held (empty), and then gradually you let the lungs inhale a minimal amount and then exhale again and hold it. As this exercise is continued, a comfortable rhythm and amount of inhalation is found which provides some wonderful feelings which open you to further experiences.

This exercise can then be reversed with filling the lungs and doing the reverse with the lungs held full with a small amount of air being released and then refilling etc. The first exercise of emptying the lungs can be added to with some of the movement and feelings of the *uddīyānī*, and similarly the *jālandhara* can be added in part to the filled lungs exercise. The addition of the movements or pressures of the *uddīyānī* and *jālandhara* to the *kumbhaka* type exercises should be done carefully with a small effort initially, and then you look for added good feelings and then change the whole program to maximize them. As you follow the increasing sense of good feelings, the body starts to change such that the body becomes capable of producing more and more *shakti* and tolerance for it.

The next level of *mahāsādhanas* develops the *kanda*. The previous *sādhanas* dealt with experiencing the inner sensations, developing the inner organs, and producing *shakti* energy from *prāna* energy. The next efforts will be to start to direct the flow of inner fluids or sexual "juices" into the *kanda* to cause it to develop and swell.

In general, whereas you have been increasing good inner feelings in the above exercises, you will now develop the control of an organ. In beginning to work with the *kanda* it is profitable to have stimulated your

189

inner feelings with the prior exercises so that your body feels very energized and sensual. Chapter Nine should be well understood with a mental picture of a swelling *kanda* in your *yoni*. It can be imagined as being very flaccid and soft but with some slight amount of swelling. You may experiment with the swelling of the *kanda* either sitting or lying flat on your back with very light finger contact which can be exploratory as well as stimulating.

If possible, stimulate your nipples or have someone else do it for you as you concentrate on a flow into your *kanda*. Do not apply too much pressure (which seems to be what is initially desired), but rather feel that you are looking for something very sensual and delicate. If nothing is experienced do not be concerned, as it may take longer to prepare the inner development, simply continue the preceding *mahāsādhanas*. Men may find it easier to find the beginning of the *kanda* since it will appear as a slight soft swelling where the base of the penis might be expected, however, the penis should not be enlarged. Women may first be confused with swelling of the labia and must look more inward to find an even softer and larger area of swelling. At this stage of development, the power of *mantra* is obvious as the mental vision obviously precedes and is so necessary for the physical manifesting of the *kanda*.

As the *kanda* swells, it becomes very sensitive to touch and when stimulated gives rise to ever increasing pleasant feelings within the body which are more systemic than local. It is no doubt this type of feeling that prompts the sitting and rocking motions of some children and adults with strong emotional feelings such as grief, frustration, laughter, etc. The massage or rubbing of the nipples further increases the systemic feelings which is also no doubt related to the hugging and caressing of the self found in grief, etc.

Once the *kanda* is found and fully activated, another sensation is found that is the urge to press the *kanda* further outward. As this sensation is explored with the model of the *Shiva linga*, an inner force is found that can in fact press outward forming a more solid protrusion from the *kanda*. As this force is applied, there is initially many times a feeling of rupturing yourself as a definite protrusion of a mass is pressed through the outer layers of the body. This protrusion of the *Shiva linga* has mental as well as global body feelings associated with it that can perhaps best be described as "opening." The opening is toward the physical world as well as the experiences taking place in the world. It is a state of awakening described in *Sanskrit* as *unmesha* or the process of opening the eyes. This opening allows you to go beyond the brain's conditioned response to the outside world and "see."

As the new organs become developed, it is noted that they swell or protrude during times of emotion, demands, or strong feelings without your effort. They become associated with the rise in "seeing" or responding to a new world.

The pleasure and the further development can be materially increased with the contact with another person's *kanda* and this is the basis for much of the misunderstanding of the *Tantrik* sexual practices.

The ritual of the *Tantriks* is found written with many variations today, but all do have much the same central common theme. Using this theme with the prior descriptions in this book, a brief description of the early practices can be described for those who would attempt to find the *Tantrik* ecstasy of ritual. The two participants of the practice are individually prepared with bath and cleansing and then come together to honor each other and the Divine. They touch, anoint and caress each other reaching for the union with the Divine in the kingdom of Heaven. This is described as the sacrificing (*ādi yāga*) of the Self to your partner and to the higher power of the union. They allow their bodies to take on the androgynous nature of the Divine and then seek physical union through their hearts or *yonis*. The woman then finds a position in the seated lap of the male (beginners may use a male reclining position) such that the *yonis* enmesh (no penis contact). The hearts open to each other and rub and entwine together in *samghatta*. This is the famous *Tantrik* ritual and *mudrā* with *samghatta*. It should also be noted that the bodies are quiet and only the interiors of the *yonis* are in motion. (Note: *ghatta* means "to rub" such as done with the *Shiva linga* icons and *sam* means "together or jointly." It does not mean to have intercourse as commonly translated.[17])

Modern experiments on this ancient practice for modern couples finds that the ancient instructions and definitions are excellent. It was found that the nipple stimulation of each other may be required to speed up the opening and activation of the *kandas* as done in the individual practices. The *samghatta* or rubbing cannot be done by a beginner, since the required muscles and responses may not be sufficiently developed in the *yoni*,

---

[17] See Table 2 in *Part F* for further variations of modern terms vs. ancient.

although the couple may supplement this weakness with some external motions. As the *kandas* become swollen, the next major step of *kunda golaka* or ball and socket interaction can be attempted.

A firm spot of one *kanda* presses into a softer area of the other *kanda* and then the muscles vibrate giving rise to further stimulation of the *Shiva linga* which then penetrates or presses deeper into the other *kanda*. This process can continue to feel better and better as more and more of the two bodies become involved in either responding to or in support of the rising ecstasy of the contact. As this proceeds, there are a number of sensations described in terms of vibrations, jumps, quivers and the ultimate indescribable vibration called *avācya* which means you become unable to describe it.

As this process is mastered the ecstasy far surpasses any found in the normal sexual intercourse and it can in fact be maintained for hours. One of the sources of ecstasy found is with the simultaneous response of both bodies that supports the concept of the *nādis* of each other becoming coupled together through the central connections in the *yonis*. The *yonis* are both the source of *soma* and the *nādis* that interconnect the *tattvas* within each body so each *yoni* drinks of the *soma* of the other as well as coupling the two sets of *tattvas* tightly together. This sensation is supported by one of the ancient names of the *yoni* that is "the lower mouth." It is no doubt the experiences of such a union that inspired the two volumes of writing in the *Rig Veda* about the superlative properties of *soma* and union. This experience should not be expected to happen immediately for beginners, but should be anticipated and yearned for.

The effect of this *maithuna* is very long lasting with the over-all result of your world becoming more alive and filled and perhaps only the poetry of the *Rig Veda* can begin to sing the praise of this state. You find increased challenges and the abilities to meet them. You find increased union with your partner and others as your empathy increases. Your feelings and senses are increased and are trusted more than your mental judgments and thoughts.

The same experiences can be obtained with individual practice without a physical partner with proper pressure on the *yoni* as has been described. With the individual practice, however, the union with an *Ishvara* is sought instead of a partner. The "Lord" is made real through *samādhi* and the same resulting flow of *soma* is found. It is no doubt this experience that

Gopi Krishna and Saint John of the Cross described.[18] Both sexes experience the feminine feeling of penetration and also the masculine effort of reaching and thrusting forward of the *Shiva linga*.

As you interact closely with others in the marketplace, you feel a similar *yoni* movement that you do in your *mahāsādhanas*, which likewise becomes more and more pleasant and your *kanda* and *Shiva linga* appear to contribute to the energy of the play. Many times, you are aware of a warmth in the *yoni* and yet at other times you become aware of the thrusting forth of the *Shiva linga*. Many times, there is no correlation between this excitation and the experiences that seems to be much like a young pubescent boy's unpredictable and uncontrollable erection. After observing the effects over a period of time, however, you become aware of the added activity of both the *Mulādhāra* and *Sahasrāra chakras* in your daily life.

The next and perhaps the most important step in these higher practices is the shaping of your role and the outer world. The new world, role or Self when standing in its own light (*samādhi*) is not a modification of or addition of your old world. Rather, it requires the expenditure of even more effort than you have used to cling to who you thought you were supposed to be in the old world. In other words, you will have to work constantly at maintaining a new you. This is because of two reasons, the first is the strong attraction for the old self. The other is that in becoming new, your world also becomes new and you must in essence start learning all over again similar to the stepping into a strange dream. You experienced these problems in the past when you attempted to break free of what you were taught that your body was supposed to be and what you were supposed to feel.

Assume that you have in fact stepped into your own future or into your new world; the battle is still not over and in fact becomes even greater. Since the change is new, it takes continual effort to remain there since the body and mind are conditioned to be with the old self and world. You have had the experience of really feeling good or of losing yourself in the moment when a small sexual thought or a doubt about the outcome of the moment leads you off into your old conditioned world.

---

[18] See Chapter 9.

The Sermon on the Mount in the Bible is based upon the problems of being in the higher state or new world. The yearning to remain there is obvious and the faith that you are in good hands or *pure in heart* is essential. Furthermore, you must obey all of the smallest requirements in the new world. A small doubt for instance or a slight irritation can send you tumbling back into the lower or older world. Jesus described this as having to follow the laws more so than the most obedient people in your old world. If in your old world you could get by with the normal level of sinning, in the new world, any sin, no matter how small can send you plummeting.

As an example of faith, you may well have experienced the situation wherein you are opening up to someone who needs help and find yourself giving some advice. Suddenly you question your "right" to offer such advice and find that you cannot continue with the same insight and authority. You might find yourself in the company of beautiful people and thoroughly overpowered with some conversation when you notice a mole on their face, or discover they have bad breath and again you are doomed to remain in the old judgmental isolated world you were taught to hang out in. The admonition of Jesus of "do not judge" is fundamental to staying in a new role.

The Christian statements about loving your enemy or not judging your fellow man describe *mahāsādhanas*. This is because only those in the kingdom of Heaven could do them, and they used these teachings to increase the *vimarsha* in their life. For others, the commandments were only more disciplines or rules that they should attempt to follow. For those people who attempt to control themselves and to be good, an enemy remains an enemy, no matter how hard they attempt to convince themselves otherwise. One common evasion that is used to satisfy and even boost their ego is to label their enemies as enemies of God, their church, their beliefs, etc. and therefore they can justify their judgement and really put even more energy into condemning them.

One practical starting point that you can use in stepping into a new world is to accept the power in the outer created world and then flow with its pace, intensity, and demands rather than your own interpretations of what it should be. It is standard for you to be impatient or desirous of time to slow down. You normally might consider yourself running to stay up with the outer world or dragging your heels in an attempt to slow it down. There is a relaxed comfortable feeling as you find the pace of the outer world, trust it, and flow with it. Similarly, you find the demands upon you either too severe or insufficient to keep you fully alive. To meet this challenge, faith in the game is required and trust that what you are called upon to do is the best. Hence, the old expression of doing your duty is a good start. It is often that you feel that the demands of life are too great and again faith in the game is required. Even if you have never faced the current problem before, if you have faith in the game and perceive it as a game, then you cannot fail even if you are hopelessly overpowered. The *Tao* has the best writings on this subject and must be understood also, as applying primarily to those in the upper world or kingdom of Heaven.

Another related problem can be equated to not having fully united the sun and Moon. It is a common feeling of having the sense of not being completely connected to the outer world. You are reacting to the world, but without full comprehension of yourself and the interactions. Many times, it may appear to be the overlapping of some other time and place on top of the immediate game. You are like the child who is attempting to play but thinking about another game, except that you may not be aware of what game or thing is interfering. What must be done is similar to the above "flowing with" as you resign yourself to that which is occurring and being experienced without judgement and with *shakti*.

As a seeker begins to be aware and review life, a general direction, theme, or path can be perceived. Perhaps, initially nothing more is felt than a deep urge to understand, to belong, to explore and create, or to excel. As you work with the practices, this deep sense of the Will can be seen more clearly and the attachment to the glitter of the conditioned world fades.

The changing that is being discussed is not at the conditioned level but rather that at the Soul or Spirit level. This changing is of the nature of freeing you from the conditioned limitations and bondages. This changing is more like returning to what you started out to do than changing to something unknown. As you review your life, one thing becomes out-standing and that is the return of the enthusiasm, drive, curiosity, learning ability, and trust you had as a young child. Compared to where you are now, this review generally causes you to wonder if you are the same person you were as a child. The goals and dedications you had as a child are vastly different from what most people have as adults. Somewhere in your life your goals shifted from learning, enjoying, experimenting and being filled with the wonderment of the vastness of the world, to the normal adult life of pleasing and using people while attempting to satisfy your desires. Above all you had to maintain your supreme importance. Most adults have desires for maintaining or increasing their status quo with little or no effort.

Once you are able to "see" the basic dedication of your life, the first awakening is that the world is perfect for the fulfillment of that dedication. The role and world are then clarified and energized. The world then becomes supportive to your dedication and every occurrence becomes a positive step whether it is a loss of a job or an award for superior service. When this goal is manifested, you can experience the continual expansion of your world and pleasure.

With the dedication of seeking and exploring, you find that you must possess super powers along the path or to be able to assume a different role. For instance, you might find yourself faced with a question which must be answered or a task which must be accomplished for which you have neither the training nor the basic skills. It is at these times that *mantra* must be used to perceive the new Self with the powers required. Then as the poet Emily Dickenson states, when "we are called to rise…our statures touch the sky."

And there is still more!

PART E

RESOURCES

Table 1 ~ The Tattvas

The following Table 1 list the *tattvas* numerically and then with an associated *Sanskrit* letter or sound. Following the name of the *tattva* is a brief description of the function, nature or power of the *tattva*, followed by one or more examples or elaboration. The **center bold divisions** list the level of the Self associated with the following *tattvas*. The **<u>underlined bold words</u>** and statements list the associated *chakras* and brief descriptions of the functioning.

Many writers assert that the sound of associated *Sanskrit* letter is related to the actual subtle feeling of the *tattva*. This may have been when *Sanskrit* was spoken since it does indeed have a strong and strange relationship between sounds and feelings. However, modern languages appear to have lost much of this power and so have the speakers of the modern languages. A further confusion also results from the use of two alphabets using different orders of letters in *Sanskrit*, so that a *tattva* would be designated by a different letter in the two systems.

Nonetheless, there are different *tattvas* and each *tattva* does indeed have a specific vibration (or a specific molecular structure.) These are coupled into a *chakra* which has two ways of responding to a similar vibration. One is from outside the Self, and the second is the projection of that vibration outward from the *chakra*. Each *chakra* therefore has the capability of either responding to a specific feeling or to generate that feeling.

The system of *chakras* is programmed by default according to one's conditioning. A new dedication can change the programming with sufficient *shakti*. The Self is the result of all of the *tattvas*—from the shape of the body, through the basic intention or purpose, to the fundamental consciousness of the Self as an individual. In order to change what you are or what you project, your *tattvas* must be changed. The *tattvas* of the total Self can therefore be equated to a summation of vibrations. This is like a sentence made up of words that are made up of a sequence of letters or sounds. If one *tattva* is changed, a word likewise changes and therefore the statement of the Self.[19]

---

[19] Table 3 lists some *Tantrik* terms of vibration.

Table 1   **The *Tattvas***

#		Name	Description	Examples
1	*a*	*Shiva*	Masculine Force	Potentiality *Entelechy*
2	*ha*	*Shakti*	Feminine Force	Energy Manifested

Pre-Spirit—*Aham*

Mulādhāra Chakra

"Smell" of life – Basis of Distinction
Cohesion—Feet—Earth

#		Name	Description	Examples
3	*s'a*	*Sadāshiva*	*Jnāna*–God	*I* am this I consciousness
4	*sha*	*Ishvara*	*Kriya*–Lord	*This* I am Distinction
5	*sa*		*Shuddhavidyā*	Pure wisdom I *am This* Definition

Spirit—*Ahamkāra*

#		Name	Description	Examples
6	*va*	*māyā*	Limiting	This is That Limitation

Svādishthāna Chakra

"Taste" of life – Basis of Will
Contraction—Hands—Water

#		Name	Description	Examples
7	*la*	*kalā*	Agency	Capability
8	*ra*	*vidyā*	Wisdom	Wisdom

Table 1 The Tattvas

9	*ya*	*rāga*	To color	Passion Intensity
10	*ma*	*purusha*	Spiritual form	Intention
11	*bha*	*prakriti*	Original form 3 *Gunas*	Feelings
12	*ba*	*buddhi*	Retaining concepts	Intellect

Manipura Chakra

"Sight" – Basis of Action
Expansion—Anus—Fire

13	*pha*	*ahamkāra*	Making by the Self	*Bhāva* Role

Soul—*Atman*

14	*pa*	*manas*	Physical mind	Control
15	*na*	*shrota*	Ear, the 9 – 11 body openings	
16	*dha*	*tvachā*	Sense of Touch	
17	*da*	*chaksu*	Eye	
18	*tha*	*rasanā*	Taste Organ	
19	*ta*	*ghrāna*	Nose	
20	*n'a*	*vāk*	Speech	
21	*dha*	*pāni*	Hand	
22	*ga*	*pāda*	Foot	

Anahata Chakra

"Touch" – Basis of Interaction
Penis—Air—Guard (*Hidden function of nipples.*)

23	*tha*	*pāyu*	Gate of *shakti*	Guard (*Hidden function of Nipples.*)

Self—*Jiva*

24	*ta*	*upastha*	Control Center	Sheltered place underneath
25	*n'a*	*shabda*	Word	
26	*jha*	*sparsha*	Touch	
27	*ja*	*rupa*	Form – Color	
28	*cha*	*rasa*	Taste	
29	*ca*	*gandha*	Smell	
30	*na*	*ākāsha*	Aether	Connections
31	*gha*	*vāyu*	Air	Separation
32	*ga*	*agni*	Fire	Energy
33	*kha*	*jala*	Water	Time-change
34	*ka*	*prithivi*	Earth	Physical stuff

Vishuddha Chakra

"Hearing"
Interaction—Aether

Table 1 The Tattvas

| 35-51 | The 16 vowels are not definitive but relate to the processes and activities in the outer world. |

Table 2 ~ Comparison of Tantrik Writings and Terms

There are two major differences between ancient and modern translations of *Tantrik* documents. The chief difference is the removal of special powers from an individual and its replacement with a dependency upon an institution or God in modern versions. Another difference is the concept of the basic physiology of men and women.

An example of the basis for the difference is in the understanding of the name of a *Tantrik* scripture called the *Rudrayāmala*. *Rudra* was described as an androgenous God and *yamala* means "coupled or paired." The combined word is called a *tatpurusha* compound in *Sanskrit* grammar in which the case or usage of the first word is lost. Therefore, the compounded word can be translated as either the union of *Rudra* or the union with *Rudra*. The first translation would be the coupling with a feminine and masculine nature or androgyny. The second would be to find a union with *Rudra* such as in worship. There is an almost identical problem with two Christian translations: the faith *of* Jesus or the faith *in* Jesus.

Additional examples of the removal of powers away from individuals is with *soma* and *kundalinī*. These two terms are accepted as meaning powers that either no longer exist or are attributed only to gods or super humans. The modern schools believe that the Western model of sex is complete and accurate, while the earlier model assumes a hidden sex in both men and women with separate organs and functions as discussed further in Chapter Nine.

A related difference in translation concerns the Five M's of *Tantra* which are assumed in modern times to describe the secret meetings of *Tantriks*. The Five "M's" or *Panchamakaras* are: *mānsa, mudrā, matsya, madya*, and *maithuna* which are commonly translated as describing a drunken (*madya*) group eating forbidden meat (*mānsa*) and fish (*matsya*) with an aphrodisiac (*mudra*) during a sex orgy (*maithuna*). The earlier meaning which is based on a literal translation of the words can mean: ecstatic, sensual, vibrant, expressive and union with each other and the Divine.

These two opposing meanings can be compared with the early Christian love feasts and the commentaries about them from their critics. The writings of an early 11th century critic, Kshemendra[20] in Kashmir may well be one of the sources of the shift in translations, as he accused the early *Tantriks* of gross obscene behavior including drunkenness and sexual rites as perhaps the least objectionable.

Tantra is built upon the knowledge that you can develop a super feminine organ with its super functions in your present body, be it male or female. This super feminine organ consists of the *yoni* and *kanda* that can be developed through special practices or *sādhanās*. The activated *yoni* becomes more pleasurable than the penis or clitoris. Men identified its placement, receptiveness and sensitivity with the vagina in females and hence referred to a *yogi* who had developed such a *yoni* as female or *yogini*.

It is also obvious that such a person with the developed *yoni* could be listed as androgenous. The ancient literature is chiefly oriented to the male, and no direct references are known that describe the results in the female. But modern studies do demonstrate the corresponding attainment of a hidden masculinity in women that comes with the development of a *Shiva linga* which swells like a penis out of the *kanda* and *yoni*.

Such a *Shiva linga* can also be an organ for experiencing intense pleasure in two modes: an urge to press it outward or an inward pulling-up sensation, *urdhva retas*. A discharge which is called *soma*, described as having very powerful properties, is associated with the *kanda* and the *Shiva linga*. The external secretion of *soma* is clear, has a silky feeling, and is absorbed rapidly through the skin.

Since modern translators with the Western view of the body could not accept that *soma* is produced internally as described in the writings of the *Rig Veda*, they naturally attempted to ascribe its production to some plant or mushroom with psychedelic properties. The early writings describing the pressing and pounding necessary to produce *soma* became then a recipe for producing *soma* from plants. In the course of history many people have attempted to discover the plants that had the wonderful properties described in the *Rig Veda*, but of course without results. This viewpoint that *soma* is produced from plants has persisted, however, thus

---

[20]https://en.wikipedia.org/wiki/Kshemendra

Table 2 ~ Comparison of Tantrik Writings and Terms

weakening the teachings of the *Rig Veda*. In actual practice the pressing and pounding takes place as a churning in the abdomen and an internal pounding of the *kanda*.

The following Table 2 on the next page lists some of the popular translations of *Tantrik* words that are given meanings obviously because of the Western physiological viewpoint. The literal meaning is also given which can provide an insight into the so-called hidden practices of *Tantra* if looked at with "eyes open."

Table 2	Comparison of *Tantrik* Writings and Terms.	
Sanskrit	**Literal**	**Popular**
acharyākrama:	to move oneself; *krama*: step-by-step	secret rites, *ādi yāga*
adrishtamandalo:	unseen creative fluid: *soma*	sacred *mandala*
ādi yāga:	primal giving or sacrifice	coitus
Sanskrit	**Literal**	**Popular**
ardhanārishvar:	androgyny: (*ardha*: two halves + *nāra*: physical self + *ishvar*: Shiva)	*Shiva*
brahmacharya:	following a Divine guidance	sex abstinence
charyāvidhhi:	*chary*: practice; *vidhi*: to pierce (*chakras*)[21]	coitus

---

[21] See *Shatchakrabheda* in the *Sanskrit Tantrik* Dictionary.

Sanskrit	Literal	Popular
guhya:	concealed, hidden (male *yoni*)	female pudenda
kanda:	bulb, 3rd sex gland, source of *shakti*	penis
kāma-kalā:	controlling pleasure	sex practices
kramamudra:	*krama*: step-by-step + *mudra*: position	coitus
kriyāmudrā:	energizing or creative posture	coitus
kulayāga:	*kula*: rite; *yā*: to proceed (with purpose); undertake; *ga*: going quickly, reacting to; (intensive ritual)	coitus
Sanskrit	**Literal**	**Popular**
kunda-golaka:	pit shaped/globe or ball (*yoni*-to-*yoni* posture)	coitus
maithuna:	paired; coupled; united	coitus
Rudro:	androgyny, *Rudra* with a feminine "o"	The God *Rudra*
Rudrayāmala:	androgyny; *Shiva* as both god and goddess (*Bhairavā* and *Bhairavi*) + *yāmala*: pair	coitus

Table 2 ~ Comparison of Tantrik Writings and Terms

samghatta:	to rub together	coitus
shākinis:	androgynous members of a *Tantrik* group	special *yogis*
shukra:	clear bright fluid; *soma* from both sexes	semen
smarānanda:	continuing bliss of quivering (as a leaf)	remembered sex
soma:	mind and body altering biochemical produced from within the body	intoxicating: mushroom juice
svayambhu:	self-made *lingam* or *Shiva linga*	inner penis
Sanskrit	**Literal**	**Popular**
taccodakah:	*soma*: radiant water or fluid	ambrosia: *amrita*
tapas:	fervor, heat	austerities
upastha:	lower center of existence; *yoni*	vagina
yoginmelaka:	female *yogi* + *melaka*: gathering[22]	mystical meeting
yoni:	male or female opening for *kanda*[23]	female sex organ

---

[22] A sacred meeting where all have the nature of female *yogis*.
[23] The opening in males covered by the perineum.

yonyarsha:	fleshy excrescence from the *yoni, kanda*	hemorrhoid of the *yoni*

Modern writings about *Tantra* speak of hidden secrets, but surprisingly, there do not appear to be major secrets. The "secret" aspects appear as *Sanskrit* words are shifted in meaning to present an image acceptable to today's world. Modern translators of the ancient texts do for the most part indicate extreme honesty in their translations, since the majority include the *Sanskrit* term after their shifting of the literal meaning.

A translator's task is to take a text from one language from one time and place and present it in another language to another time and place such that it is understandable.

In today's world it is assumed that men do not have female organs and that sex can only be performed by penetration of the vulva with a penis. Modern Academia has made broad declarations of what constitutes the basic physiological processes as well as the methodology of interactions of people. *Tantra* does, however, point to other processes and physiologies as can be evidenced by a comparison of some of the critical *Sanskrit* terms.

Sanskrit scholars were aware of the problem of translating texts and report two methods of translating the ancient writings. One method is to follow the literal or original interpretation, *pratishabdam*, while the other is to read in the context of experience or what appears reasonable or meaningful, *yathsambhavam*.

Table 3 ~ Tantrik Terms of Vibration

Vibration or *spanda* is used to describe the manifested sensations associated with the rise of *shakti* and *kundalinī*. These vibrations can be experienced in a wide variety of ways depending upon the intensity of the rising energy, the immediate demands upon the body and mind as well as the dedication.

In general, the very forceful inner thumpings, poundings, jumps are connected with the beginning of the rise of *kundalinī* or the production of *soma*. The intoxicating swirling types of vibrations that still allow the functioning in the outer world are indications of the changes in the body caused by the inner energy or *soma*.

For instance, many people when facing a crisis feel overwhelmed with their world spinning and then remember nothing as they react unexpectedly to some crisis and then undergo some supernormal response. The shaking or throwing off vibrations are indications of the dedication overriding the conditioned doubts and fears of the brain and body. The churning and throbbing sensations are generally results of increasing the *shakti* energy. The remaining types of vibrations should be obvious and are generally related to the interaction with the outer world or to *maithuna*.

Table 3	*Tantrik* **Terms of Vibration**
1.	*abhigāta*: striking against
2.	*abhigharshana*: rubbing against, friction against
3.	*avadhuta*: to shake off (opposing forces, blockages, or sins)[24]
4.	*bhrama*: to roam, whirl, flutter
5.	*bhramavega*: to whirl, flutter with intense energy and rate
6.	*chalana*: slow vibration
7.	*chalattā*: tremor (as of sudden relaxation)
8.	*chandah*: harmony

---

[24] See *dadhyāshirā*.

9. *dadhyāshirā*: conduit of shaking down
10. *dhvani*: audible sound, vibrant resonances, implied meanings
11. *gurni*: intense vibration with dizziness, intoxication
12. *kala*: low tone, murmur
13. *kampa*: trembling
14. *kampana*: medium rate vibration
15. *kinchichalana*: subtle unmanifested vibrations
16. *kshoba* = *kshubh*: to tremble, to shake, agitated, stir up
17. *lalanā*: to sport or play, tongue, caress or cherish, radiant or quivering
18. *lalita*: amorous, quivering, tremulous, languid gesture, lolling
19. *madya*: intoxicating, exhilarating
20. *mantham*: churning
21. *matsya*: like a fish
22. *matsyodari*: pulsating like a fish
23. *mocana*: releasing from, discharging
24. *nāda*: inner sound, tinnitus
25. *nāddanta*: directed *nāda*
26. *pipīlika*: ant, like an ant, tingling
27. *pranava*: *pranu*: to roar, reverberate; sacred sound, *Om*
28. *shabda*: sound, the cognizing of *artha* (or *nāma*)
29. *smarānanda*: continuing bliss of quivering (as a leaf)
30. *spanda*: quivering, throbbing as of life
31. *spandana*: fast rate vibration

Table 2 ~ Comparison of Tantrik Writings and Terms

32. **sphota**: bursting forth, creative sounds
33. **sphur**: to spring, tremble, throb, break forth, to live
34. **ubdha**: jump
35. **unmanā**: mental excitement, perplexity, facing the unknown
36. **visarga**: emission, expansion, "more"
37. **vishuvat**: *vi-shu* + *vat*: to surround: equinox, center of forces

Table 4 ~ The Parātrimshikā

Table 4   *The Parātrimshikā*

1. *Devi* asks *Deva*:

   How can *Tantrik* powers quickly open the kingdom of Heaven with the knowledge of *mātrena* that opens the path to Heaven?

   Tell me of this hidden aspect of myself which shines forth largely unhidden.

2. Tell me, *Deva*, about that *Tantrik* power that resides in the *hridaya* as the ruling feminine power of the body, (and tell me) in what way can I find fulfillment?

3. The illustrious feminine power is the source of great Divine gifts in the kingdom of Heaven.

4. By maintaining *Tantrik* practices, the desired world is made real, thrust forth from the Heaven within your heart (*hridaya*). I am revealing to you the powers of the kingdom of Heaven.

5. Now! We begin with: all of the reality of Heaven can be found to be built on and becomes manifest with the subtle union of the Moon and Sun.

6. The physical or manifest is in union with the creative force in the evolving world. Evolution proceeds step-by-step from one realm to another, as the letter "*Ka*" to the letter "*Ma*."

7. There are four supporting elements of reality: air, fire, flowing water, and manifested earth. From these there arises a shining forth proceeding the developing of the expansive world.

8. Without beginning, they are the steps of bringing forth all that is known, experienced, and created. Everything is truly *mantra*, knowledge, and glorious.

9. This *yoni* is filled with the "shining forth" of the four illustrious elements in balance with the expansive world.

10. The third nature of *Brahma*, or the *hridaya* between the thighs, unites the Soul with the Divine. Those who do not have the existence as a *yogini* or the state of androgyny, as did the god *Rudra*, cannot break forth.

11. This *hridaya* is the dwelling place of the God of Gods and is the source of union with liberation at the same time. Ascending (beyond) is accomplished with the uniting of the great *mantra* and *mudrā*.

12. At the moment of opening, the body moves expressing the union with a continuing expression and enjoyment of sensual and ecstatic up-flowing feelings associated with a *mudrā*.

13. At that time, one attains the empirical form of the *mantra-mudrā*, which was created in the future and becomes manifest in the present.

14. The thoughts can be thrust forward into time by the androgynous power of *Rudra* to make a clearly manifest and real spiritual shining form.

15. The thrusting forth of *mantra* and *mudrā* with pure consciousness brings forth complete true knowledge and the higher powers of the *yogi* (masculine).

16. The inner great masculine power directs and sets in motion the coming together of the creative powers.

Table 4 ~ The Parātriṃshikā

17. The inner perceptive powerful drive results in the obtaining of *mantra* and the power over the faultless manifest.

18. The junction of the two *Tantrik* powers brings forth all of the powers in the form of a flowing unseen creative fluid (*soma*).

19. The unseen fertile fluid moves, and thus, with this motion, reality is known, a portion of his powers come into their own existence, *he* is a *yogi* (feminine), he is also initiated.

20. Being blameless and with the knowledge of *mātrena*, he knows all of the powers (*shaktis*). Even without the training of *yoga*, he becomes one with the assembly of *shākinis*.

21. However, without knowing the rules, he brings forth worship.

22. The manifested world is first begun with *mātrena*, then shaped with *māyā*. The masculine force pervades the boundless created world with its three mentally created powers of spiritual creation, destruction, and maintenance.

23. The inner continual process of life becomes a pure path for the one who perseveres in the rules. It quickly opens to the knowledge of the inner sovereign powers.

24. Because of the radiant fluid (*soma*) one is a great Soul, knowing the masculine powers of *Shiva* and all things. One is without sin, one's will and exertions become pure and shining.

25. As the great banyan tree is contained within the energy of its seed, so also is the evolutionary upper "kingdom of Heaven" contained as a seed in the *hridaya*.

26. Truly, bound with the knowledge of the true state, the reaching for oblivion (*nirvāna*) fades away, dedication comes into existence;

doubts, anointings and impressive religious ceremonies are abandoned.

27. Having made the object of worship manifest and united with that seed, the goal is reached.

28. The inner seed bursts forward as the Moon becomes full, coming forth from the inner lotus of the heart meditation with *soma* exerting one's own security.

29. Whatever is desired and made a dedication to becomes reality. The power of knowing all is not reached for but rather abides within.

30. This manifested *mantra* bursts forth from the combined masculine and feminine powers to attain all knowledge and powers.

Table 5 ~ The Sermon on the Mount According to Tantra

Table 5	The Sermon on the Mount According to *Tantra*

1. Jesus, on beholding the large gathering of people looking for miracles, retreated to a private spot with his disciples who were starting to experience the kingdom of Heaven and desired to know more.

2. He opened to the inner creative power and spoke as if from on high.

3. When you can trust and yield to the higher power then you can remain in the kingdom of Heaven.

4. In the kingdom of Heaven you will have grief, but with that grief comes both relief and gain.

5. With humility you can obtain anything you are dedicated to.

6. When you find the balance (righteousness) of the masculine and feminine powers within yourself, then you will be filled with the spirit and divine energy.

7. You will find your self filled with tenderness, but the world will also appear to be tender.

8. When you find the purity and clarity of the mind then you will gaze with amazement upon the higher power.

9. When the world around you becomes at oneness, then you will be considered the reflection of the higher power.

10. When you find others reacting strongly against you, then this, too, is the kingdom of Heaven.

11. When there are those who would harm you in any way and pervert your teachings and statements, then the inner spirit is strong.

12. When these happen, then rejoice and know that you follow the path of ecstasy trodden by many saints before you.

13. You have the potential for changing the earth, but if you ignore the potential, then you indeed find death.

14. You have an inner light and you must reach your summit so that it can shine from there and illumine the darkness and be seen.

15. Is this not the same as putting a candle high on a holder so that it illumes the whole room?

16. As you follow your dedication, people will see your great works and marvel at your inner creative power.

17. Do not consider that I oppose the World of Law or Mammon, but rather that I teach of going beyond.

18. The outer laws of society will remain until all can master them and find the inner power.

19. Anyone who breaks or teaches breaking any laws of society is far from the kingdom of Heaven; whoever teaches and supports the laws is opening to the kingdom of Heaven.

20. But for you who wish to enter the kingdom of Heaven, you must be able to obey every aspect of the required law even more so than those representing the laws.

21. The law states that no one may kill and if one does, he shall be held accountable to the court of law,

22. but the requirements for those residing in the kingdom of Heaven are that you may not be even be angry or perceive foolishness in those close to you or you will find the return to the judgmental state of the lower world.

23. If you wish to find purity in mind, but feel a remembrance that someone was hurt because of your actions,

24. you must first make amends and then seek the purity.

Table 5 ~ The Sermon on the Mount According to Tantra

25. The adversarial statements arising in your mind must be addressed instantly while you are able to resolve them and before you condemn yourself and fall into the prison of self-pity and hopelessness.

26. Once you fall into self-condemnation, every contributing remembrance must be resolved and renounced.

27. You have been taught that it is wrong to commit sexual violations,

28. but in the kingdom of Heaven, even the thoughts associated with lusting remove you back to the World of Law.

29. You must renounce any single observation of the outer world that binds you to continual self-judgment or else your whole being remains bound to the lower world.

30. You must renounce any action that you do or have done that binds you to continual self-judgement or else your whole being remains locked in the lower world.

31. The law states that you can be separated from your spouse,

32. but you are guilty of sexual violation if this is not done solely because of the dedication and bonding of your spouse to someone else.

33. The law states that any oath must be properly witnessed and recorded,

34. but you should not give an oath or promise based upon the will of the Divine,

35. nor upon the earth, or any place for they are all the place of the Divine,

36. nor should you swear upon your own will for you cannot even control your own hairs.

37. You will rather simply state your intentions with a yes or a no.

38. The law entitles you to seek an eye for an eye or a tooth for tooth when damaged,

39. but the kingdom of Heaven requires the acceptance of being damaged and further that you support that which is occurring.

40. If someone in your upper world has power to take one of your possessions, then offer your other possessions.

41. If someone asks you to give them the results of your effort, then give them more than what they ask to fully comply with the demands of the upper kingdom.

42. Respond fully to the requests of those with you in the upper world and do not resist anything.

43. Everyone is taught to love their neighbor and hate their enemy,

44. but in the upper world, you must love those who oppose or harm you and support them that speak against you and encourage those who use you to further their own actions even if they disparage you.

45. This is so that you may be as a child responding fully to the game presided over by the inner power. This inner power is coupled with the same power that provides the setting for the game of life for everyone.

46. How can you find joy if you have only those who love you in your game of life? Isn't this what those in the lower social World of Law desire?

47. If you honor and support only your close friends, is this not also a characteristic of the lower world of suffering?

48. You must therefore become outwardly as perfect as the Divine power dwelling within you.

PART F

APPENDIX

Appendix A ~ Response Time for Tantriks

A simple experiment was performed with a group of people who had been practicing some of the advanced practices of *Yoga* in terms of their reaction time. This experiment was devised to prove that those who practice advanced *Yoga* have a much quicker response time which when coupled with *jnāna* explains why the martial arts came forth from the early schools of *Yoga*.

A measurement of the time it took a group of middle-aged people using the prescribed *sādhanās* to respond to the sound of a clap was compared with a control group of about the same average age and a group of children. The test required keeping the eyes closed to avoid any visual clues and keeping their hands at their side to equalize the required distance to move the hands and then to clap the hands as soon as possible following the sound of a clap. A sound engineer analyzed a sound recording to evaluate the actual time of response.

The two control groups consisted of a group of 18 children, 12 to 13 years old and a group of 14 middle-aged men and women. Two times were measured, one for the fastest individual response and the second for the time between the first and the last clap or the time interval of the groups response which gave an indication of the uniformity of the group's response.

This study is quite exciting since it indicates that practices counter the normal drop off in response time with aging with for instance the conclusion that a seventy-year-old *Tantrik* student had a response time faster than an average 12-year-old. It also shows that the average response time takes twice as long for people of about the same age not engaged in the ancient practices.

Response Time for *Tantriks*

Time in seconds	*Tantriks*	12-13 year-olds	Adults
Fastest Time	0.170	0.240	0.320
Time Interval	0.110	0.140	0.250
Average Time	0.225	0.310	0.445
Slowest Time	0.280	0.380	0.570

Appendix B ~ The Greatest Medical Myth

The Greatest Medical Myth is that Medicine increases the length of life. A secondary myth is that the miracle drugs of medicine have worked miracles.

Perhaps the best example of the fear tactics being used to sell medical services is that which is currently being used with breast cancer. The common quote is that one woman in nine or over 11% of all women will develop cancer of the breast. This data is true if you are 85 years old, but the actual data needs to be reviewed. Fortunately, the statistics of death are readily available with the easiest source being given in the Almanacs. The first questions to be answered are what are people actually dying of and how many are dying? The following table is an abbreviation of a government listing with the graphical presentation given in Figure 1.

If you are concerned about dying, then according to statistics you should be exercising and watching your diet, since that accounts for the decrease in heart disease shown above, and heart disease is over six times more likely to cause your death than breast cancer. The rise in breast cancer can be attributed to the decrease in the mobility and movement of the breast and nipple as exemplified in women wearing wire-supported bras and sleeping bras. The other obvious statement that can be made about any cancer is that cancer is primarily an old age disease and everyone must die of something as will be discussed next.

The remaining issue is that the medical ads imply that if you get properly diagnosed then you will be cured of the cancer, but there is again no data to support this implied claim since cancer deaths continue to climb despite more aggressive treatments. If there were a positive treatment it should be apparent in the curves of Figure 1, demonstrating a rapid drop in fatalities which is the graph of the above data.

Figure 2 presents the death rate data for the U.S. since 1900 and is primarily interesting for the upward rise during the flu (pneumonia) epidemic of the 1910's and then for the absence of any major variations after that. One would have expected to find a rapid drop off in death rates with the introduction of the miracle drugs starting in the 1940's. The major downward trend of the curve dominates which is explained by the increase of sanitation and improvement in the diet of the average American. The curve demonstrates that the garbage collector and greengrocer have contributed more to the life expectancy of the nation than has the doctor or pharmacist.

Another curve is given in Figure 3 that shows the rise in life expectancy broken down by age groups. For a newborn baby the life expectancy has increased from about 28 years in 1850 to about seventy years in 1990. Again, this increase is due to the garbage collector, window screens, sewers, etc. Similarly, no great sudden increase is noted for any of the groups during the 1940's and on.

In summary, there is definite concrete data showing that taking care of your sanitation, exercise, and diet can increase your life to some extent; however, there is no evidence that surgery or pills will change the average life expectancy. The key word here is "average" and this requires discrimination when it comes to purchased medical treatment even if you believe that it is only your health insurance that is paying the bill.

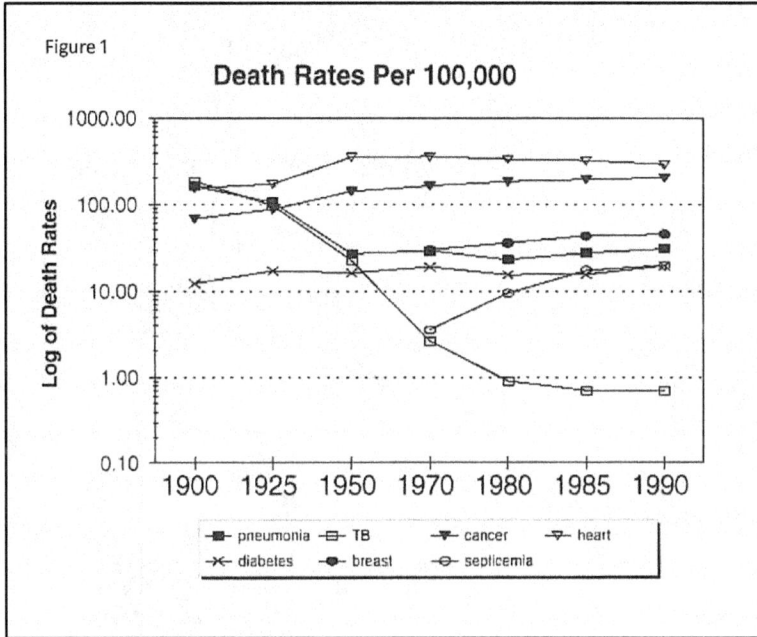

Figure 1

Death Rates Per 100,000

This data and its graph (Figure 1.) show the more or less constant trend of illnesses in the United States. Tuberculosis (TB), for instance, was dropping at a constant rate before the introduction of the antibiotics. Cancer, on the other hand, remains relatively constant despite the major introduction of intensive treatments.

Death Rates Per 100,000

Cause of Death	1900	1925	1950	1970	1980	1985	1990
Heart Disease	153	170	358	362	336	323	289
Cancers	68	87	140	163	184	193	202
Breast Cancer				30	36	40	45
Pneumonia	162	105	27	31	24	28	31
Diabetes	12	17	16	19	15	16	20
Septicemia				2	4	7	8
TB	185	97	23	3	1	.7	.7
All Causes	1621	1157	960	950	880	870	860

Figure 2.

Death Rate All Causes

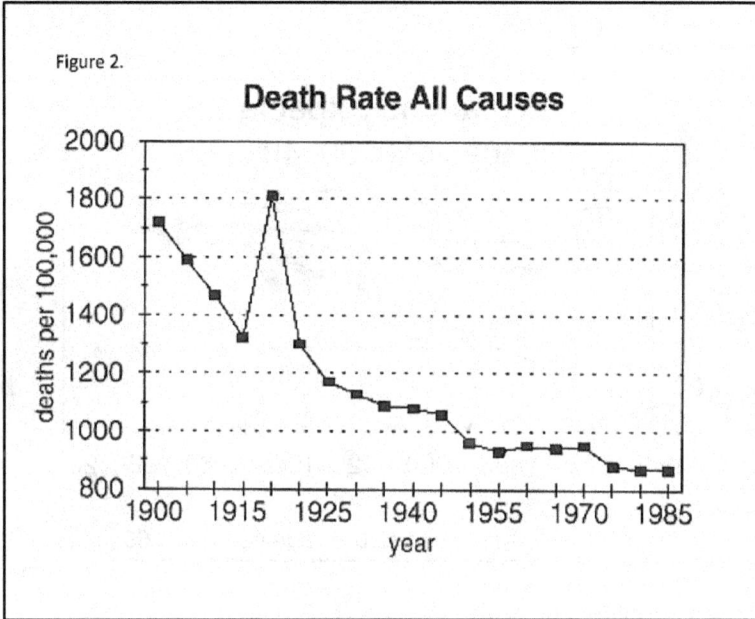

This graph (Figure 2.) demonstrates the gradual reduction in the death rate since 1900. The sharp rise in the curve demonstrates its sensitivity, since that peak was the result of the famous flu epidemic of the 1900's. This curve, like the other two, does not demonstrate any sharp decrease in death rates after the introduction of the "miracle drugs" or "advanced surgical procedures."

Figure 3

Total Life Expectancy
for ages of 0, 20, 40 and 60

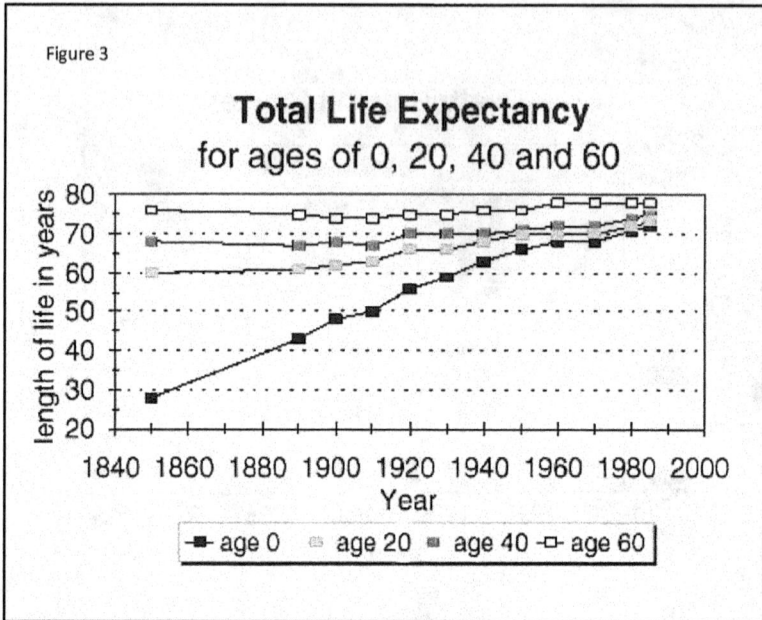

length of life in years

80
70
60
50
40
30
20

1840 1860 1880 1900 1920 1940 1960 1980 2000

Year

—■— age 0   ▨ age 20   ▪ age 40   -□- age 60

This graph (Figure 3.) demonstrates the remarkable increase in the life expectancy for people of differing age groups. The increase in longevity is seen to be fairly uniform starting in the 1850's. The decrease in death rates is very easy to attribute to the increase in hygienic practices as well as an increase in food diversity and quantity. This curve gives direct evidence of the importance of civil engineers, farmers, truckers, and sanitation workers to the increase in life expectancy. There is no direct evidence, on the other hand, of any contribution from the very expensive medical profession which should have demonstrated a rapid drop starting in the late 1940's with the advent of the miracle drugs and intensive medical treatments.

Appendix C ~ References

The following listing is based upon availability or importance to the interpretations presented in this book. The fundamental *Sanskrit Yoga* texts are the *Yoga* of Patanjali, the *Hathayogapradipika* and *Paratrishika-Vivarana*. These texts are obscure, allegorical, and require an experience of the content before full understanding can be obtained. There are a number of translations available of these writings, but they all vary considerably in terms of translations. The cited texts of the *Hathayoga-pradipika* and *Paratrishika-Vivarana* include the original *Sanskrit* that may be of assistance to the serious student.

Energy
> Peck, R., Peck, T., The Stone of the Philosophers, 1988, Personal Development Center

Hermaphrodites
> Fausto-Sterling, Anne, The Five Sexes, The Sciences, New York Academy of Science, March/April 1993

Kingdom of Heaven (God)
> Liderbach, Daniel, The numinous Universe, 1989, Paulist Press

Mantra
> Singh, Jaideva, *Paratrishika-Vivarana*, 1988, Motilal Banarsidass

Tantra and Yoga
> Dasgupta, Bhushan, Tantric Buddhism, 1974, Shambala
>
> Dyczkowski, M., Doctrine of Vibration, 1987, SUNY
>
> Krishna, Gopi, Kundalini, 1967, Shambala
>
> Mishra, K., Kashmir Saivism, 1993 Rudra Press
>
> Mishra, R. The Textbook of Yoga Psychology, 1987, Julian Press
>
> Peck, R., Peck T., The Philosophy of Patanjali, 1994, Personal Development Center

Peck, R. American Meditation and Beginning Yoga, 1976, Personal Development Center

Peck, R., Peck, T., Kundalini, Sex and Yoga, 1989, Academy of Religion and Psychic Research

Silburn, L., *Kundalini*, 1988, SUNY

Svatmarama, *Hathayogapradipika*, 1972, Theosophical Society

Woodroffe, John, The Serpent Power, 1974, Ganesh & Co.

Appendix D ~ Sanskrit Tantrik Dictionary

The following list on page 237 gives the *Sanskrit* word in *italics* followed by its closest rendering to the usage in this book, *The Golden Triangle*.

The meaning of the root may be given for clarification and similarly for prefixes, suffixes or the merger of different words. One interesting feature of many of the compound words used in *Tantrik* texts is that the meaning of a compound word is the sum of all of the combinations of possible word groupings.

In some cases, the popularly accepted or used meaning of a *Sanskrit* term will be given in square brackets [ ] if it disagrees with the original or literal usage.

Sanskrit (*Tantrik*) -to-English Dictionary

—A—

a: (as a prefix to a word) negation, not

abhaya: not fearful, security

abhi: towards, approaching

abhidā: literal power of a word, to set forth

abhigāta: striking against

abhigharshana: rubbing against, friction against

abhinava: *abhi*: to approach, *nava*: new, fresh

abhipreta: intention, to approach with the mind

ac: to, towards

accha: transparent, clear

ad: to eat

ādhi: to be over, above

ādhibhautika: *adhi* + *bhu*, control of what is becoming

ādhidaivika: *ādhi* + *deva*, Divine power of the physical realm, game or life

adhishthāna: to stand over, to empower, to overpower

adhyātma: the supreme self

ādi: the beginning

ādi yāga: primal giving or sacrifice

adrshtamandalo: *adrsht*: unseen; *manda*: cream, spirituous liquid: *anda*: egg, semen, unseen creative fluid

adya: now, food

ādya: to be eaten

āgan: to attain, arrive, reach

āgama: approaching, traditional concepts, scripture

agni: fire, the god of fire

āgni: referring to *agni*

aham: "I", Spirit behind Soul and Self

ahamkāra: conditioned self: *Aham* + *kāra*: action

ahimsā: respect of others, non-harmful

aishvara: from a power, lord

ahu: to sacrifice (religious), oblation

āj: to drive towards, (to bring forth)

ājnā: 6th *chakra*, command, perceive, understand, unlimited power

akasha: ether, space

ākrishtam: drawn, pulled toward one's Self, to call forth for a spirit

amarolī: the controlled taking of urine

amrita: immortal, spiritous liquor, ambrosia, *soma*: a fluid offering supernatural powers.

amula: without beginning

anāhata: 4th *chakra*, living; *an*: move, *ana*: breathe, *hath*: to force

ānanda: bliss, beatitude

ananta: eternal, boundless

anāshrita: unmanifested, detached

ānava upāya: *ānava*: belonging to men, humane; *upāya*: means, arrival

ānava mala: sins of Man

anena: without fault

anta: end, limit

antar: within

ānta: final

anu: fine, minute

anugraha: revealing
essential nature

anuttara: chief, supreme
reality, external world is the
internal, kingdom of Heaven

antahkarana: inner mind
(*karana*: doing, making)

apa: water, air, intermediate
region, river

apāna: downward air flow

aparā: not remote or
beyond, the past

api: to enter in, partake,
join

ardhanārishvara: *arha*:
two halves; *nāri*: male;
ishvara: *Durga*, Goddess; half
man-half goddess or female

artha: meaning, object,
thing, purpose, wealth

as: to reach, arrive at,
obtain

āsana: sitting in a particular
manner, control of the lower
body, posturing.

āshram(a): dwelling place
of the *guru*, teaching center; a
stage of life

ashtānga yoga: consists of
yama, *niyama*, *āsana*,
prānayāma, *pratyāhāra*,
dhāranā, *dhyāna* and *samādhi*

asta: thrown, given up

asteya: respect of property
of others, non-stealing

at: to roam, attain

athā: now!

ātman: the Soul of Man;
the manifesting of life

aum: sound of the *nadam*,
inner sound, cosmic sound

aunmukyha: expectancy

avabhāsa: radiating light or
splendor, radiant appearance

avācya: not describable

avap: to reach, obtain

avidyā: not knowledge,
nescience, wisdom in
opposition to truth

—B—

bala: strength, power

bandha: a tightly locked
āsana or *mudra*

bhadrā: auspicious, good

bhaga: enjoyment

bhāga: allotment,
inheritance, luck

bhakti: devotee of love

bhautika: elemental-
material

bhava: coming into
existence, being

bhāva: becoming,
appearance, state of being
anything

bhāvanā: causing to be,
producing, imagination

bhaya: fear

bheda: stimulating

bhoga: enjoyment of sense
objects

bhuta: *bhu*: to become

bhuvana: a being, a place
of being

bīja: seed

bimba: an object for
comparison, source,

image, reflection

bindhu: seed, luminous dot
at *ajna*

Brahmā: the Creator, God

brahmacharya: *Brahma*:
the Divine power; *charya*: the
path of; [no sex]

Brahma(n): the God within
yourself, *Īshvara*

bhrama: to roam, whirl,
flutter

bhramavega: to whirl,
flutter with intense
energy and rate

buddhi: the power of
forming and retaining
conceptions and general
notions, intellect

—C—

car: to move into, pervade

catur: four

charvanā: perceptive,
experiencing with delight

chakra: wheel or circle;
interfacing organ between
gross and subtle; group of
intimate people practicing
Tantra

chchanda: pleasing,
alluring

chchandas: desire, will

chā: concealing

chalana: slow vibration

chalattā: tremor, as of
sudden relaxation

chandah: harmony

chandra: glittering, moon,
soma, water

chara: moving, movable

chari: to move, walk, live,

busy with, conduct one's Self,
a path

charyāvidhhi: practice;
vidhi: to pierce (*chakras*) (See
shatchakrabheda.)

chira: a long time

chit: consciousness,
awareness,
individuality

chumbaka: one who kisses
much, sensual

—D—

dabh: to hurt, deceive,
destroy

dadhyāshirā: conduit of
shaking down; *da*: producing,
dhā: to take hold of, *dhu*: to
shake down, *dadhi*: curds and
whey (from churning); *sira*:
vein-like channel; [to serve
soma with curds]

daksha: expert, capable,
industrious, intelligent

dakshinacharga: the path
of perfecting, right-hand path

dasā: states

deha: to shape or form,
body, form

deva: divine, heavenly, god

Deva: the inner abiding
masculine Divine force, Lord,
Shiva

Devī: The inner abiding
feminine Divine force, Lady,
Shakti

dhāranā: holding or
maintaining (a fixed world),
concentration

dharma: permanent or

Divine law, one's state of
perfection

dhvani: audible sound,
vibrant resonances, implied
meanings

dhyā: to think, meditate on

dhyāna: control of
thoughts, meditation

digdha: soiled, anointed

dīksha: initiation, complete
dedication resignation to

div; *diva*: heaven with three
levels, lower, middle and
upper (*uttara*) vaults

druma: tree

dukha: uneasy, pain,
sorrow

dva: two, two genders, both

dvaita: two, dual, duality

dyā: to attack, assail

—E—

esh: glide or hasten towards

evam: in this way

—G—

gam: to go, towards or
away, to send, to move
forward in time, to change
state, denote

gāmin: going, moving on,
in or towards, reaching to

gandha: smell; *ishta*: good;
anishta: bad; *madhura*: sweet;
katu: pungent-stimulating;
nirhārin: diffusively fragrant-
coming out; *samhata*:
complex; *snigdha*: smooth-
oily; *ruksha*: dry-harsh;
vishada: pure-soft

garbha: womb

gav: desirous, wishing

gava: cow, the cow as a
symbol for higher
consciousness etc. (See *go*.)

gāvah: cow, radiance of
sun, higher consciousness,
source of *ghi* or *ghrita*

gavāsirā: channel of
seeking (literal: channel of
seeking cows); [*soma* served
with milk]

ghatt: to rub, to shake or
stir up

ghi: clarified butter, mental
or spiritual clarity of mind

ghora: awful, terrible;
mahaghoras: inner demons or
negative forces

ghrita: (See *ghi*.)

go: cow; of a cow; the stars
(See *gava*.)

golaka: ball (See *kunda-
golaka*.) [for sexual
intercourse]

granthi: to tie together, a
knot, an inner obstacle to
shakti

gupta: *gup*: protect, hide

gurni: intense vibration
with dizziness, intoxication

guha: hiding place

guhya: concealed, hidden;
yoni or *kanda*; [sex organs]

—H—

hā: to leave, discharge,
remove, avoid, be left behind

hi: to send forth, impel,
hasten on

hiranya-garbha: golden;

garbha: the interior, a womb; the golden interior or womb

hri: to take, carry, bring, offer, appropriate (legally), overpower, interact

hridaya: "heart," source or center of life or activity (not vital organ); *yoni, hri*: + *day*: to possess, partake; (center) of interaction

hridayam: *yoni ūpam*: *yoni*; *ūpam*: towards, near to, resemblance; heart

—I—

ichā (*ichchhā*): desire, inclination, long for, intention

ichā mrityu: power to die at will

idā: animation, vital spirit, chief left *nādī* of heating or masculine nature

Indra: to conquer, god of sky, inner power of conquest fed from *soma*

Indu: a drop: *soma*, moon, phases of moon

indriya: of the outer senses

ish: to endeavor to obtain, to yearn for (See *ichā*.)

īsh: to rule, obtain, seek

īshtra: the protecting Divine force; *īsh*: to rule; *ish*: to yearn for; *tra*: to protect

īshvara: a ruling deity or power; *ish*: to yearn for; *īsh*: to rule, the personal ruling God or Lord, *Brahma*

Īshvara pranidhana:

Īshvara: ruling God; *pranidhāna*: receptive of leadership

ishyamāna: *yama*: restraint, curbing; narrowing down the desire to a specific desire

—J—

jālandhara: a *bandha* of pushing up *prāna* to the head

janani: mother, (*jan*: to create)

jāti: genus or class

jāyā: bringing forth, a wife

jihva: tongue, tongue of *Agni*, tongue of fire, upward flow of *shakti*

jīva: the total self, role, ego

jnā: to know (as *gnosis*), perceive, remember

jnāna: higher knowledge, *gnosis*, mental creation, visualization, Truth

jnānendriya: knowing or awareness of subtle forces in outer world

jnānendriyani: state of knowing

jneya: to be known, to be learnt

jyā: to overpower, oppress

—K—

kala: low tone, murmur

kalā: a single part, agency, *kal*: to incite, Divine or higher power

kāla: black, hidden, subtle; *Shiva*: power of the Divine; *kāl*: to count, hence time *kālāgnim*: dark-sun, dark-light, unmanifest/manifest

kalasha: a water pot, a churn, a woman's breasts

kālayogin: ruling over

kalpanā: mental composing/creating

kam: to wish for, desire

kāma: wish, desire, pleasure, longing for

kāma-kalā: controlling pleasure (with upper and lower *chakras*)

kāmayate: dedicated to

kampa: trembling

kampana: medium rate vibration

kanchukas: constrictors time (*kāla*), attachment (*rajā*), space (*niyati*), knowledge (*vidyā*), agency (*kalā*)

kanda: (*yonyarshas*) swollen fleshy protrusion from *yoni*, source of *shakti*; [collapsed uterus, base of penis]

karana: act or means of doing, cause

kārana: cause of anything

karmendriya: effecting the outer world, the outward projection of inner feelings

karuna: mournful, lamenting, compassionate, pity

kārya: action, the created, effect

kath: to tell, show, command

katham: question of "how", in what manner?

kaula: union with those who evolved to the level of *vāmachāra* or beyond, member of a *Tantrik* group.

Kaulachāra: path of Oneness with world, freedom

kaulika: related to *kaula*, *Tantrik* follower

kaulikasiddhidam: liberating powers gained through *Tantrik* practices

kha: opening, heaven

khechari: *kha-chari*: the path of the sky, kingdom of Heaven, or higher plane

khyā: known, proclaimed

kosha: sheath

krama: in regular order, step-by-step

kramamudra: ordered position, ordered *nimīlana* and *unnimīlana* (eyes opened closed); expansion to contraction; [sexual intercourse]

krita: done, made, accomplished

kritvan: causing

kriyā: to create, undertake, do

krodha: anger, passion, wrath (envy, hatred, oppression etc.

Kshā: the earth, ground

kshānta: endured, experienced

kshana: view, sight, to foretell

kshoba: = *kshubh*: to tremble, to shake, agitated, stir up, stirring joy *kula*: related to *Kāli*, of *Tantra*, totality, supreme energy of *Siva*, solidification (consciousness)

kulayāga: *kula*: rite; *kula*: energy, *yā*: to proceed (with purpose), undertake; *ga*: going quickly, reacting to; [sexual intercourse]

kumbhaka: breath retention, being as a pot

kunda: pot-shaped, hole containing coals and fire

kunda-golaka: *kunda*: bowl-shape; *golaka*: ball-shaped; *Tantrik* union (ball and socket, junction of *yonis*; [sexual intercourse]

kundala: ring, fetter, coil as of a coiled rope

kundalin: decorated with earrings, a snake, energy of transcendence

kundalinī: transformational energy

—L—

labh: to catch, gain possession of

lakshana: expressing indirectly, symbol

lakshana: *lakshanā trayam*: the three levels of meaning of a word: historical, modified and combinations

lalanā: to sport or play, tongue, caress or cherish, radiant or quivering

lalita: amorous, quivering tremulous, languid gesture, lolling

laya: to cling to, to disappear, destruction, spiritual indifference

līlā: absorption in play, like child's game, oneness or *maithuna* with activities of life

lo: of a man

—M—

ma: letter "M"; I or me; moon

mā: to measure, show, exhibit, (See *mātrā*.); negation

madya: intoxicating, exhilarating, ecstatic; [being drunk with wine]

mad-yama: controlled madness or exhilaration.

madhu: the drink of the Gods

madhyamā: middle, intermediate

maithuna-gamana: *maithuna* + *gamana*: to approach carnally; sexual intercourse.

mahā: great

mahābhāga: the great share or portion

mahā-bandha: A *mudra* combining the *jālandhara* with tightening the *yoni* muscles

mahābhuta: elements of physical reality: earth, air, fire and water, ether

mahālīlā: the sacred, higher, future games that humans can aspire to.

mahāmudrā: the

experienced world and Self become reflective of one *mudrā*.

mahāsādhanas: advanced disciplines for reaching for perfection

mahā-vedha: a *mudra* combining the *mahā-bandha* with banging the *yoni* against the ground

maithuna: (*mith*: union as friends or enemies); (*mithuna*: paired, twins); coupled, union, state of oneness with each other; [copulation]

mala: dirt/filth, original sin, sin; *mala-ānava*: conditioned sins;
   -*mā -yiya*: from separation; -*kārma*: from own actions

mama: me, myself, mine

manas: mind

mand: rejoice, intoxicated; pause

maṇḍa: cream, spirituous liquid

manda: moving slowly

mandala: circular, circular drawing

manipura: 3rd *chakra*, filling of desire; (*māni*: thinking of possessing or being) (*man*: to believe) (*pura*: filling)

mānsa: flesh, sensual; [eating meat in *Tantrik* ritual]

mantham: churning

mantra: to create mentally; *man*: brain function; *tra*: protecting; the conative process, continual mental creation, bringing together

mantrāmudrā: to make a shared total world as reflective of one purpose, feeling or *mudrā*; a world or role (*mudra*) formed with a *mantra*

mārga: seeking, path, way

mata: thought, imagined

māta: composed, made, mother

mati: devotion, prayer, intention, resolution

mātrena: *mā*: to prepare, exhibit, display, *tra*: to bring together; *mantra* and *mudra*

matta: excited with joy, intoxicated

mātrā: measure, true knowledge

Mātrika: a *Sanskrit* alphabet in which the letters are arranged phonetically as opposed to the *Mālinī* system

matsya: fish, vibrant (lower abdominal rapid vibration like a fish); [eating fish in ritual]

matsyodari: pulsating like a fish.

māyā: illusion, super natural power, veiling, creating

me: to barter, exchange

milana: eyes (*up-* opening eyes; *sam-* closing)

mīna: Pisces, the sign of the zodiac

moha: loss of consciousness, bewilderment, delusion, darkness

moksha: liberation

mudrā: sign, activate with

name or sign, a posture, body
language, a role; [eating an
aphrodisiac (fried grain) in
Tantrik ritual]

mudrita: a *mudra*,
tensioning

muhurta: a moment of
time, instant

mukha: face, countenance,
mouth

mulādhāra: 1st *chakra*, root
support, (*mula*: root, *dhāra*:
supporting)

—N—

na, *nā*: not, no

nādam: inner sound;
[tinnitus or ringing of the ears]

nādādanta: point of *nāda*;
danta: point, as a tusk

nādī: tube (subtle nerve
conduits), connections
between *tattvas*

nam: to bow, submit to,
turn towards

nāma: to name, name,
characteristic of

nah: to bind

nara: the empirical being, a
man

nava: new

nāyaka: leader, chief,
leading example

nāyikā: ruling female or
lady heroine

nimīlana: eyes opened

nir: out, without

nirvāna: oblivion; *nir*: out;
vā: to blow; [Union with the
Divine]

nirvikalpa: without mental
variations, indeterminate
consciousness, no thoughts
and awake

nirvish: to enter into

nispanda: no motion, no
spanda

nitya: one's own, eternal

nivritti: to turn inward or
back (toward spiritual)

niyama: no physical
constraint, spiritual laws
or restraints

niyagrodha: banyan tree
(growing downward)

niyati: space restriction,
fixed order restraints

nu, *nū*: to praise, shout,
thunder

nyas, *nyāsa*: to place
within, plant, insert, to
stimulate a location of the
body

—O—

ojas: power, energy, vitality
(converts to *virya*) (from
ugra)

—P—

pach: to prepare food,
offerings, the world; to
develop

pancha: (from *pach*) an
offering, the completed world;
five (5)

panchamakara: (Five M's)
madya, *mānsa*, *matsya*,
mudrā, *maithuna*
(intoxication, flesh, vibration,
posturing, union); [drunken

sex orgy with eating of meat, fish and aphrodisiacs]

parā: beyond, highest, the immediate unfolding moment

parātrimshikā: the supreme thirty (*shlokas*)

parātrīshikā: the supreme triads (Will, Knowledge, Creative Activity etc. etc.)

parashabda: causal stress

para-vāk: causal stress

pashyanti: *pashya*: seeing (non-physical), right understanding

pāyu: protecting powers or guard; gate for control of *shakti*; [anus]

phal: to burst open, seed, consequence, result of, the point

pi: to go move (See *pyāy*.)

pingala: golden colored, the chief right *nāḍī*, the cooling or feminine nature

pipīlika: ant, like an ant, tingling

pīthas: *pītha*: seat; *pitta*: bilious humour also with *vāyu* and *kapha*

prabho: shine forth

prahara: to thrust forward

praharati: to offer praise, move forward, throw

prākāmya: power of viewing the world as a play or *līlā*

prakāshā: illuminating consciousness, cosmic stress; *pra*: coming forth from: *kāsha*: becoming visible; *kāshi*: shining

prakīrtiti: revealed, announced

prakriti: physical gross manifestation, the created, physical world

prāna: *pra*: forth; *an*: to breath; vital breath, energy of creation

pranava: *pranu*: preceding the new; to roar, reverberate; sacred sound, *Om*: and/or *pra*: in front of; *nava*: new (*mātrās* of: *A,U,M, bindu, ardhachandra, nirodha, nāda, nādādanta, shakti, vyāpini, samana, unmanā*)

prānayāma: control of the vital breath or *shakti*

prasamkhyāna: *gnosis*, intuitive knowledge

prati: near, upon, towards, opposite, in comparison

pratibhā: opposite to reality, indeterminate consciousness

pratibimba: opposite nature of image; *prati*: near, comparison

pratishabdam: reading in order of the words (See *Yathāsambhavam*.)

pratyāhāra: withdrawal, rearrange, restore (of senses)

pratyaya: going toward the object (*artha*) of the mind, with certainty, apprehension, expectation

pravritti: turning outward (toward the physical world)

prayatna: effort

preta: departed, dead – spirit of dead

prishta: asked, inquired, demanded, wished for

prithvī: earth (from *pri*: to bring out of, deliver, protect)

purusha: spiritual, unmanifested created world, the creative force

pyai or *pyāy*: to swell, overflow, to be exuberant

—R—

rāga: to color or dye, passion; *rā*: to bestow, *ga*: *maithuna*, moving quickly; *gā*: to obtain

rajas: to be animated, vital energy

rajā: attachment

rajas: attribute of being energized or activated

rasa: sap, taste, character of, feeling; *shringāra*: love, *vīra*: heroism, *bībhatsa*: disgust, *raudra*: anger, *hāsya*: mirth, *bhayānaka*: terror, *karuna*: pity, wonder, *shānta*: peace, *vātsalya*: parental fondness

rata: pleased, loved, enjoyment of love

rataguru: husband

ravecarī: *ravi*: sun, *cari*: path,

retas: a flow or stream, flow of semen

rita: met with, proper, suitable, divine law, truth

rī: to set free, flow

rudrayāmala: androgyny,

Rudra: male-female God; *yāmala*: pair; dialogue between *Bhairavā* and *Bhairavī*; [sexual union in *Tantrik* ritual]

rūpa: figure, form, appearance

—S—

sa: 3rd person pronoun, junction with

sā: giving

sādhana: practices, the physical or mental means of reaching a spiritual goal

sādhaya: to make hard, firm

sadyah: promptly, at that moment, spontaneously

sākshat: with one's own eyes, clearly, in bodily form

sahāra: renunciation or dissolution (*samhāra*)

sahasrāra: 7th *chakra* (thousand spoked), *sa*: junction; *saha*: jointly; *sra*: to flow, to come from; *ra*: acquiring, heat, love, brightness; *sahasra*: a thousand

sam: junction, with, together

samādhi: joining with

samaj: to bring together, to bring into conflict, to overcome. *sam*: together or uniting; *ja*: to drive, generally the reaching for union with another person

samāj: coming together in

one accord or equality. *sam*:
together; *jā*: to drive together

samana: at one time, in one
place, here and now

samanvita: connected with,
endowed with, full of

samarpana: *sam*: with,
together; *arpana*: delivering or
handing everything over

samatā: sameness

samayam datva: coming
together, *datta*: given; [*Tantrik*
sexual intercourse]

samghatta: *sam*: together,
junction; *ghatt*: to rub over,
shake, to stir around;
[*Tantrik* coitus]

samkalpa: *sam*: completely;
klrip: come into
existence, dedication,
determination

samhāra: renunciation;
sam: together; *hāra*: removal,
taking away (also *laya*)

samhi: to strive, wish for

samhita: to unite

samsiddha: self-found
Tantrik powers

samskāras: the connection
of past experience with the
present

samvid: to know
thoroughly, perception,
consciousness

samyama: holding together,
control, concentration,
suppression

samyan: united, together

san: to gain, possess

Sanskrit: *Sáṃskṛita*:
perfected (language)

santosha: contented, good

self-image

sarva: everything, all

sat: state of (only) being

sattā: existence

sattva: essence of spirit or
purity

setu: bondage

shabda: sound, the
cognizing of *artha* (or *nāma*)

shaivachāra: path of *Shiva*
the God

shākinī: powerful, friendly
females, androgynous
members of a *Tantrik* group

shakti: mystical
transforming energy, a
Goddess of the feminine or
manifest (See *utsāha*.)

shākta: relating to *shakti*

sham: to toil at, exert
oneself, to finish, remove

shāmbhava: coming forth
from origin or *Shiva* element

shānti: from *sham*: to be at
peace; the state of union
without judgement, peace

shāntodita: *shānto*:
quiescent state versus *udita*:
emergent or awakened state

shastra: theory

shatchakrabheda: piercing
(opening) six *chakras*

shaucha: pure in body and
mind

shaya: sleeping, abiding

shi: to grant, auspiciousness

Shiva: auspicious, God of
creation-destruction, half-
male/half-female, dark

Shiva linga: A fleshy
protrusion formed out of the
swollen *kanda* with its base in

the *svādhishthāna chakra*,
source of *kundalinī*;
[imaginary inner organ]

Shivo shaktitrayam: three
powers of *Shiva*: creation,
destruction, sustenance

shloka: a maxim, terse
statement

shrina: illustrious
knowledge

shrishti: manifestation,
created (See *srishti.*)

shu: swiftly; to go

shuchi: shining, glowing

shuddha: clean, pure,
blameless

shuddhavidyā: pure
wisdom

shukra: clear fluid, *soma*;
[semen]

shukra-shonita: the
merger, mixing and absorption
of
soma; [semen and menstrual
blood]

shūnyatā: void,
unsubstantiality, beyond
human thought

siddhi: fulfillment,
entelechy, unusual power,
powers of those ahead of you

siddhantachāra: path of
perfecting actions, thoughts,
feelings

siddhāsana: an *āsana*
sitting cross-legged with one
heel against the *yoni* and the
other above the sex organ

smara: remembrance

smarānanda: *sma*: ever,
continuing; *rāna*: murmuring,
leaf; *ananda*: bliss

soma: transforming and
transcendent nectar from
kanda, moon fluid, *amrita*,
holy spirit, *kundalinī*;
[psychedelic juice obtained
from plants or mushrooms]

spanda: vibration,
quivering, throbbing as in life

spandolikā: rocking to and
fro

spandana: fast rate
vibration

sparsha: sense of touch,
feeling

sphota: bursting forth,
expansive, creative sound or
vehicle

sphur: to spring, tremble,
throb, break forth, to live

srishti: **shru**: to flow forth,
issue from, creation (also
utpatti: birth, arising)

stan: to resound

stana: female breast,
nipples of chest

sthā: to stand

sthiti: abiding, sustenance

sthula: gross

su: to go, move, good,
excellent

sukha: comfort, pleasure;
su: good, much, very;
kha: of the sky

sukshma: subtle

sushroni: *su*: to press out;
shoni: hips (beautiful hips)

sushumnā: a subtle duct
leading from the *mulādhāra* to
the *sahasrāra chakra*

sushupti, svapna, and
jāgrat: deep sleep, dreaming,
waking

249

Suresha: a god

sūrya: sun, heat, light, manifest

suvrata: religious student, very religious, ruling well

sva: own, one's own

svādhishthāna: 2nd *chakra*; to hold one's own place, (*sva*: one's own, *dhi*: to hold, *sthā*: to stand)

svādhyāya: *svā*: self; *dhyāna*: to think, imagine and to make real

svar, svarā: sunlight, bright space or sky, heaven (as sky only)

svātantrya: *sva*: self, *tantra*: rule; being ruled by *līlā* of choice

svātantryashakti: freedom + energy; independent or fundamental inner energy

svātmasamvitti: inner self (*samvitti*: perception, feeling)

svāyambhu linga: self-made controlling *lingam* (penis-like), resting place of *kundalinī*

svacchas: crystalline clear

sya: pronoun, 3rd person

—T—

taccodakah: radiant water or fluid, *soma*

taijasa: consisting of light, passionate, vigour

tam: to gasp for breath

tāma: anxiety, distress

tamas: darkness, attribute of inertia or mass, the physical stuff of the world.

tanmatra: *tan*: to radiate: *tad*: that, *mā*: to measure: *shabda*: sound, *sparsha*: touch, *rupa*: sight, *rasa*: taste, smell; ether, air, fire, water, earth

tad: he, she, it, that, this

tadanta: coming to an end by that

Tantra: *tan*: to radiate, to make manifest and *tra*: to protect, collect or form together, philosophy and practices leading to higher realm or *līlā*

tantrikas: followers of *Tantra*

tantrya: depending upon

tapas: fervor, heat; [religious practices or austerities]

tas: to fade away, to throw down

tasya: its; *tas* + *ya*; *tasya*: fallen away, lost

tāra: carrying across, saviour, radiant, shrill note

tat: that, the unknown that (See *tad*.)

tatsparsha-kshetre: *sparsha kshetra*: place of origin, fertile

tathā: in that manner

tattva: basic characteristic of something, thatness or thisness, true state, reality

tejas: sharp, brilliance, fiery energy, mystical energy

til: to anoint

tithi: 15th day of lunar

cycle, day of dividing or
separation (dark and light)

tithimadhya: middle of the
lunar day, half moon, half
dark/half light

tra: three, trinity, protector

traya: threefold

trika: trinity

trikona: three corners or
triangle

tripta: satiated, satisfied

trishika: three pointed as
trident

triloka: three worlds

trip: become satiated or
pleased

tu: to have strength

tur: to press forward,
conquering

turīya: 4ᵗʰ state of being, in
the kingdom of Heaven

— U —

ubdha: jump

ucchar: to ascend, to
empty, to utter

udāri: to set up, declare,
bring forth

udāhrita: declared, called

udāna: the upward flowing
spiritual and vitalizing energy
of the body, *ud*: up

uddīyānī: a *bandha* of
pulling up the abdominal
region

udyoga: perseverance,
exertion

unmanā: mental
excitement, perplexity, facing
the unknown

unmesha: open the eyes,

higher realm

unnimīlana: eyes closed

upa: towards, approach

upādhi: attribute

upastha: lower center of
existence, *upa*: under, down;
sthā: to stand firmly; sheltered
place, a lower substrate;
[female generative organ]

upāya: means, arrival

ūrdhva kundalinī: upward
flowing *soma* (power) within
the body

ūrdhva retas: upward
flowing *soma* [sex fluid]
within the body

utsāha: strength of will,
strenuous and continuous
exertion, power, energy

uttara: higher, superior

— V —

vaidik: related to *Veda*
scripture

vaikharī: speech

Vaishnavacāra: path of
Vishnu the God of sustaining

vajra: lightning bolt,
sudden instant motion

vajroli: a *mudra* for
developing inner abdominal
muscles, described in
symbolic images

vāk: the Word, the creative or
descriptive aspect
associated with objects

vāma: beautiful,
pleasurable, beautiful woman

vāmachāra: "left hand

251

path", the path of pleasure and beauty; [path of sexual intercourse]

varga: group

varjita: abandoned

varnas: letters

varta: subsistence

varti: conduct, treatment of; wrapping, swelling

varya: chosen, chief

vastu: really existing, plot, pith of anything

vay: to go

vaya: food, energy (mind and body), vigorous age

ve: to weave, join together

Veda: knowledge, religious writings: (*Rigveda, Yajurveda, Sāmaveda, Atharvaveda*)

vedi: an altar, usually female shaped, therefore: the waist of a woman

vena: longing, desire, care, eager, anxious

vedachara: path of law

vetti: one who knows, a sage

vidh: to worship, to be bereft

vidhi: the manifested world

vidhva: to pervade, whole, omnipresent, awareness of gross body

vidyā: knowledge, science

vidyānām: *vidyā*: knowledge, *nāma*: named or called: defining knowledge

vijna: to discern, to understand

vijnāta: discerned, known

vi: two parts

vikalpa: to choose, judge, options; *vi*: two parts, apart; *kalpa*: competent, determination

vilaya: veiling essential nature

vimarsha: the working toward a continual climaxing of *lilā, vimrish*: to touch or experience (mentally), experience as *shakti = aham* and *idam* (I and This), the object of experience

vināpi: without

vind: finding

visarga: emission, expansion, more

vishesha: distinction, individuality, substance of special kind

vishlesha: loosening, separation of lovers

vishuddha: 5th *chakra*, reaching out (*vishu*: in various directions, *vi-shu*: to press out)

vishuvat: *vishu* + *vat*: to surround: equinox, center of forces

vishva: to pervade, whole, omnipresent

virā: masculine force, *Shiva* power

virāt: *chit* associated with created whole

virya: virility, valour (See *ojas*.) [semen]

vraj: to go, move

vyakti: particulars

vyāpini: pervading or interactive energy

vyashti: separated, "the physical self"

vyavasthita: placed in order, settled, persevering in

vyoman: heaven, as air, aether

vyomasto: being in the sky, heaven

—Y—

ya: one who goes; as a suffix: the state of, result of, etc.

yā: to go, move, proceed, march

yad: which, whatever

yadva: the mind, perception

yaj: to worship

yajanam: *yaj* + *nam*: observe worship

yajna: to sacrifice (self) or reach toward the unknown, worship

yam: to sustain, support, restrain

yama: constraint: social laws

yamala: paired, twins, doubled

yantra: instrument for holding, binding

yantur: ruler, guide

yashasvin: magnificent, illustrious, glorious

yasta: entrusted, deposited

yastu: up-flowing

yat: to stretch, join, to conform with; undertaking which

yatkinchit: continual process of life

yathā: in which manner, in order that

yatana: exertion

yathāsambhavam: translating according to fact (See *pratishabdam*.)

yavāsirā: channel of aversion, *yava*: warding off, *yu*: to push toward (*āsir*: to mix together, *sirā*: a stream; [*soma* served with barley]

yena: by whom, which way; in which direction?

yo, yu; to unite, to separate

Yoga: yoked, the practice of Patanjali, a supernatural means

Yogin(n): being connected, a male follower of *yoga*, having superhuman powers

yoginī: female *yogi*, perfected *yogi* (androgenous)

yoni: female sex organ, origin, source, home, *hridaya* heart; the middle of the perineum, the lower mouth

yonyarshas: fleshy excrescence from the *yoni*, *kanda*

yukti: union with higher principle

yut: keeping off; to shine

Index

www.ingramcontent.com/pod-product-compliance
Lightning Source LLC
Chambersburg PA
CBHW070800280326
41934CB00012B/2996